The Vibrant Alkaline Soups Recipes for Busy People

Amazing On a Budget Recipes for Incredible Soups and Get Back in Shape

Bella Francis

contained within this document, including, but not limited to, — errors, omissions, or inaccuracies.

Table of contents

Creamy Avocado-Broccoli Soup

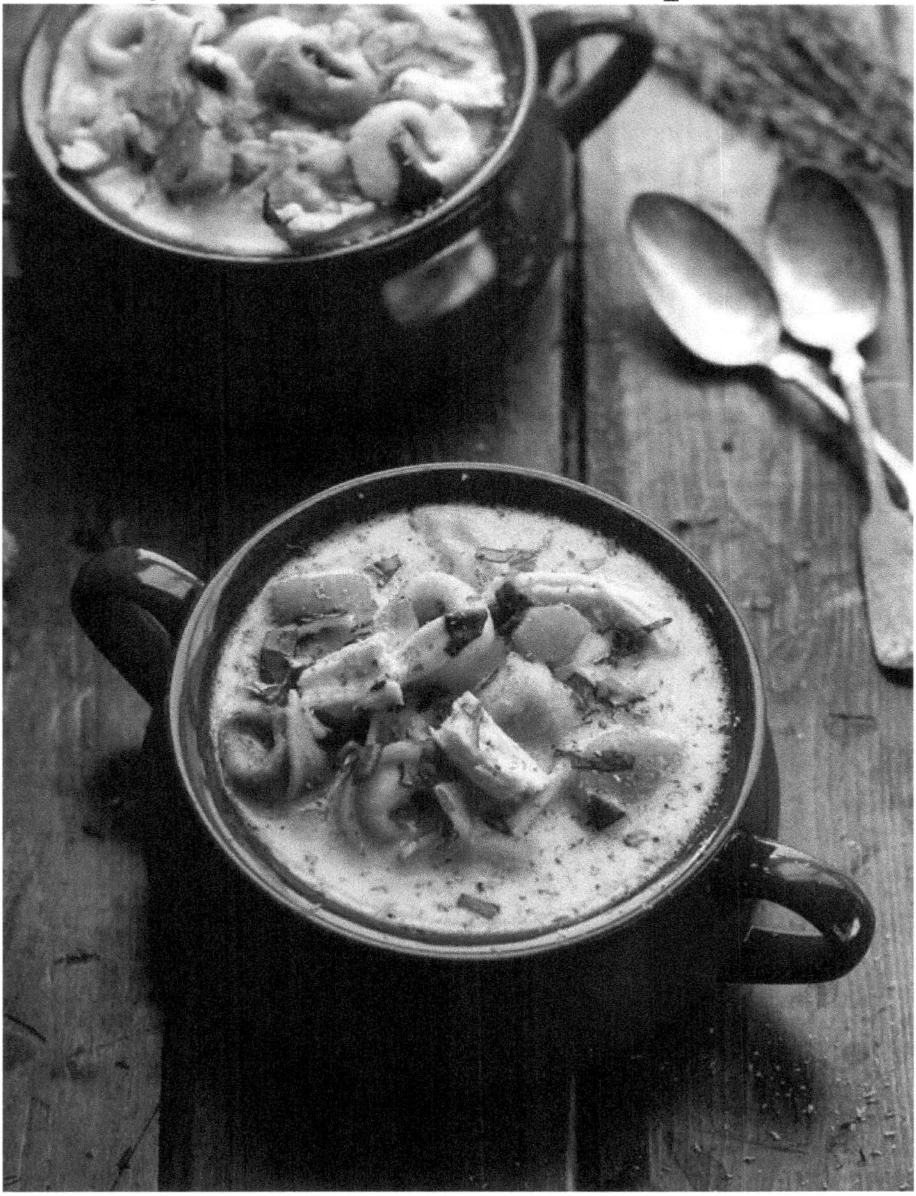

Preparation Time: 10 minutes

Cooking Time: 15 minutes

Servings: 1-2

Ingredients :

• 2-3 flowers broccoli

• 1 small avocado

• 1 yellow onion

• 1 green or red pepper

• 1 celery stalk

• 2 cups vegetable broth (yeast-free)

• Celtic Sea Salt to taste

Directions:

1. Warmth vegetable stock (don't bubble). Include hacked onion and broccoli, and warm for a few minutes. At that point put in blender, include the avocado, pepper and celery and Blend until the soup is smooth (include some more water whenever wanted). Flavor and serve warm. Delicious!!

Nutrition:

Calories: 60g

Carbohydrates: 11g

Fat: 2 g

Protein: 2g

Fresh Garden Vegetable Soup

Preparation Time: 7 minutes

Cooking Time: 20 minutes

Servings: 1-2

Ingredients :

- 2 huge carrots
- 1 little zucchini
- 1 celery stem
- 1 cup of broccoli
- 3 stalks of asparagus
- 1 yellow onion
- 1 quart of (antacid) water
- 4-5 tsps. Of sans yeast vegetable stock
- 1 tsp. new basil
- 2 tsps. Ocean salt to taste

Directions:

1. Put water in pot, include the vegetable stock just as the onion and bring to bubble.

2. In the meantime, cleave the zucchini, the broccoli and the asparagus, and shred the carrots and the celery stem in a food processor.

3. When the water is bubbling, it would be ideal if you turn off the oven as we would prefer not to heat up the vegetables. Simply put them all in the high temp water and hold up until the vegetables arrive at wanted delicacy.

4. Permit to cool somewhat, at that point put all fixings into blender and blend until you get a thick, smooth consistency.

Nutrition:

Calories: 43

Carbohydrates: 7g

Fat: 1 g

Swiss Cauliflower-Emmenthal-Soup

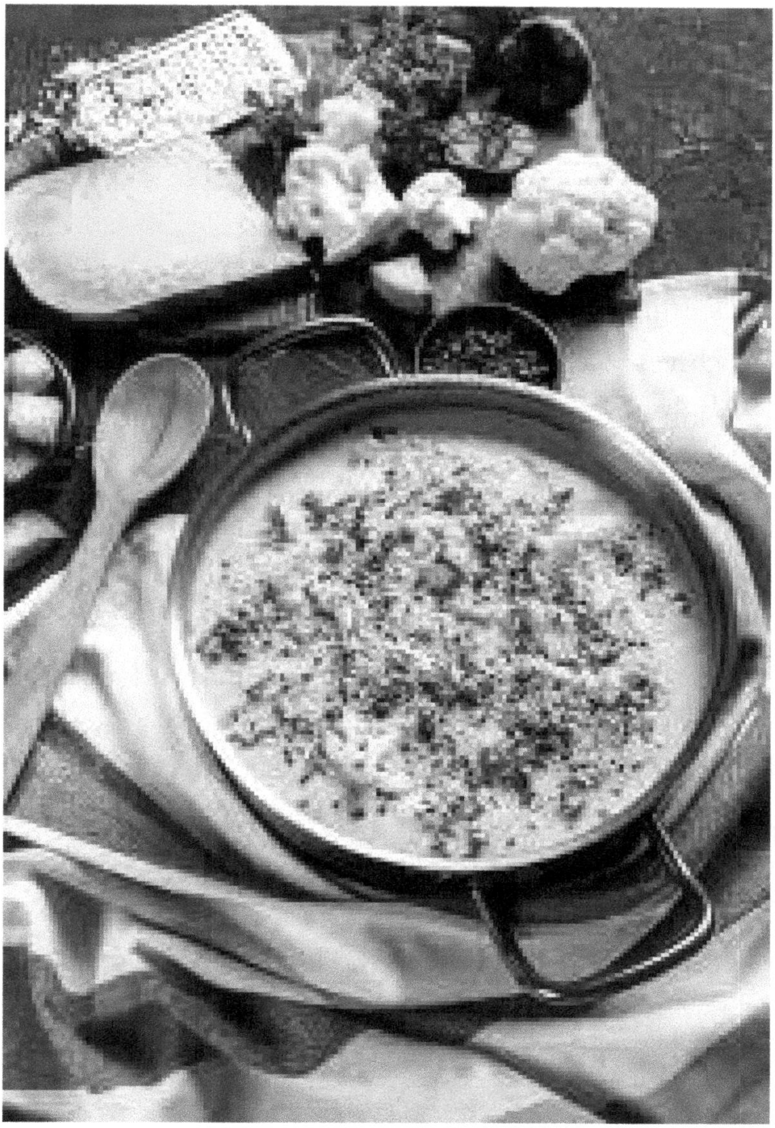

Preparation Time: 10 minutes

Cooking Time: 15 minutes

Servings: 3-4

Ingredients :

- 2 cups cauliflower pieces
- 1 cup potatoes, cubed
- 2 cups vegetables stock (without yeast)
- 3 tbsp. Swiss Emmenthal cheddar, cubed
- 2 tbsp. new chives
- 1 tbsp. pumpkin seeds
- 1 touch of nutmeg and cayenne pepper

Directions:

1. Cook cauliflower and potato in vegetable stock until delicate and Blend with a blender.

2. Season the soup with nutmeg and cayenne, and possibly somewhat salt and pepper.

3. Include emmenthal cheddar and chives and mix a couple of moments until the soup is smooth and prepared to serve. Enhance it with pumpkin seeds.

Nutrition:

Calories: 65

Carbohydrates: 13g

Fat: 2g

Protein: 1g

Lemon-Tarragon Soup

Preparation Time: 10 minutes

Cooking Time: 10 minutes

Servings: 1-2

Cashews and coconut milk replace heavy cream in this healthy version of lemon-tarragon soup, balanced by tart freshly squeezed lemon juice and fragrant tarragon. It's a light, airy soup that you won't want to miss.

Ingredients :

- 1 tablespoon avocado oil
- ½ cup diced onion
- 3 garlic cloves, crushed
- ¼ plus ⅛ teaspoon sea salt
- ¼ plus ⅛ teaspoon freshly ground black pepper
- 1 (13.5-ounce) can full-fat coconut milk
- 1 tablespoon freshly squeezed lemon juice
- ½ cup raw cashews
- 1 celery stalk
- 2 tablespoons chopped fresh tarragon

Directions:

1. In a medium skillet over medium-high warmth, heat the avocado oil. Add the onion, garlic, salt, and pepper, and sauté for 3 to 5 minutes or until the onion is soft.

2. In a high-speed blender, blend together the coconut milk, lemon juice, cashews, celery, and tarragon with the onion mixture until smooth. Adjust seasonings, if necessary.

3. Fill 1 huge or 2 little dishes and enjoy immediately, or transfer to a medium saucepan and warm on low heat for 3 to 5 minutes before serving.

Nutrition:

Calories: 60

Carbohydrates: 13 g

Protein: 0.8 g

Chilled Cucumber And Lime Soup

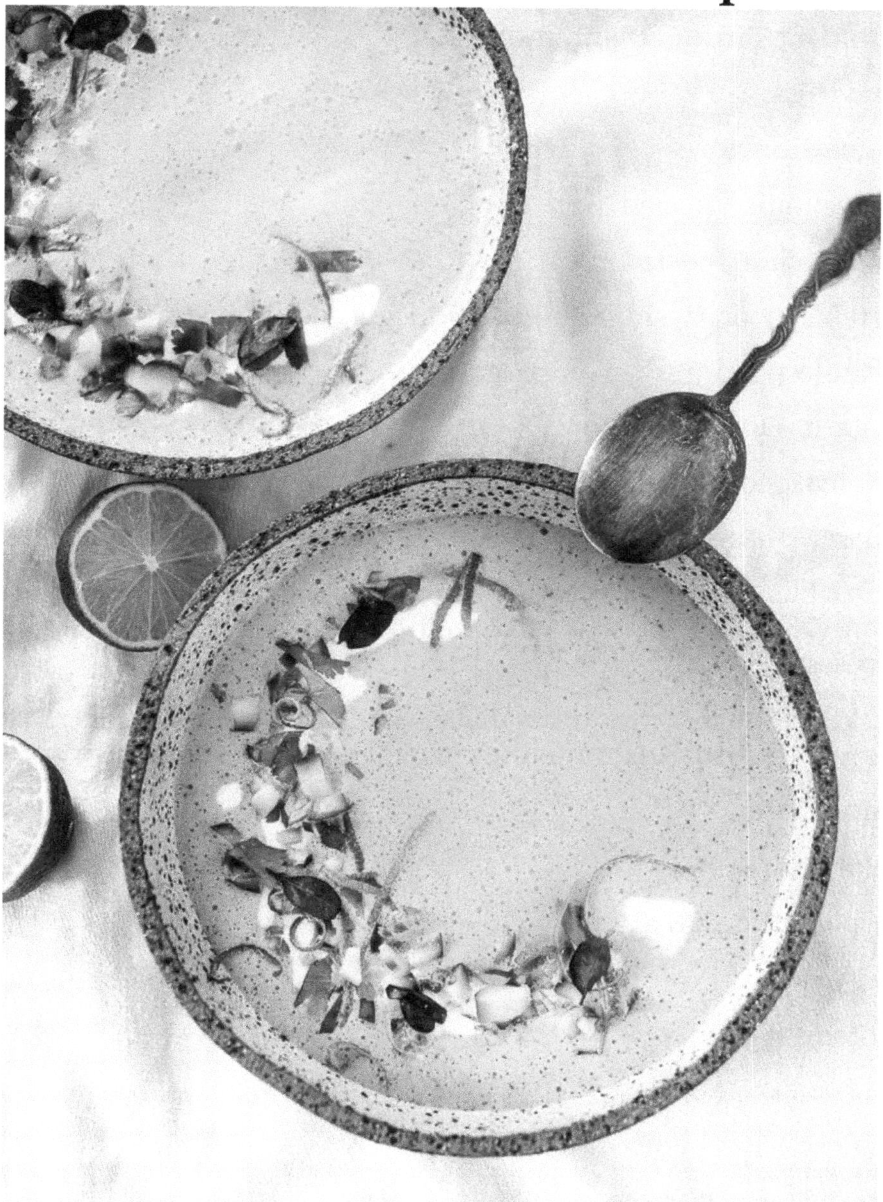

Preparation Time: 5 minutes

Cooking Time: 20 minutes

Servings: 1-2

Ingredients :

- 1 cucumber, peeled
- ½ zucchini, peeled
- 1 tablespoon freshly squeezed lime juice
- 1 tablespoon fresh cilantro leaves
- 1 garlic clove, crushed
- ¼ teaspoon sea salt

Directions:

1. In a blender, blend together the cucumber, zucchini, lime juice, cilantro, garlic, and salt until well combined. Add more salt, if necessary.

2. Fill 1 huge or 2 little dishes and enjoy immediately, or refrigerate for 15 to 20 minutes to chill before serving.

Nutrition:

Calories: 48

Carbohydrates: 8 g

Fat: 1g

Protein: .5g

Coconut, Cilantro, And Jalapeño Soup

Preparation Time: 5 minutes

Cooking Time: 5 minutes

Servings: 1-2

This soup is a nutrient dream. Cilantro is a natural anti-inflammatory and is also excellent for detoxification. And one single jalapeño has an entire day's worth of vitamin C!

Ingredients :

- 2 tablespoons avocado oil
- ½ cup diced onions
- 3 garlic cloves, crushed
- ¼ teaspoon sea salt
- 1 (13.5-ounce) can full-fat coconut milk
- 1 tablespoon freshly squeezed lime juice
- ½ to 1 jalapeño
- 2 tablespoons fresh cilantro leaves

Directions:

1. In a medium skillet over medium-high warmth, heat the avocado oil. Include the garlic, onion salt, and pepper, and sauté for 3 to 5 minutes, or until the onions are soft.

2. In a blender, blend together the coconut milk, lime juice, jalapeño, and cilantro with the onion mixture until creamy.

3. Fill 1 huge or 2 little dishes and enjoy.

Nutrition:

Calories: 75

Carbohydrates: 13 g

Fat: 2 g

Protein: 4 g

Spicy Watermelon Gazpacho

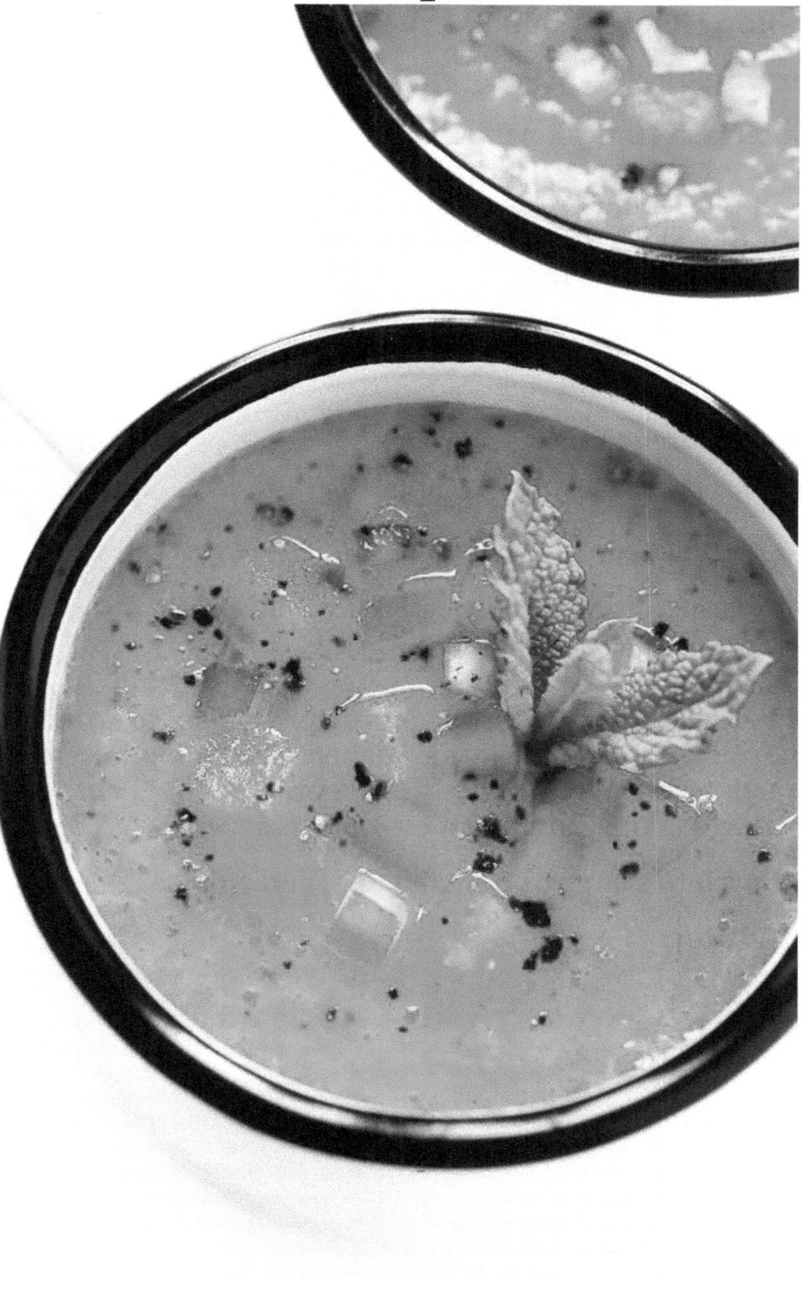

Preparation Time: 5 minutes

Cooking Time: 5 minutes

Servings: 1-2

At first taste, this soup may have you wondering if you're lunching on a hot and spicy salsa. It has the heat and seasonings of a traditional tomato-based salsa, but it also has a faint sweetness from the cool watermelon. The soup is really hot with a whole jalapeño, so if you don't like food too hot, just use half a jalapeño.

Ingredients :

- 2 cups cubed watermelon
- ¼ cup diced onion
- ¼ cup packed cilantro leaves
- ½ to 1 jalapeño
- 2 tablespoons freshly squeezed lime juice

Directions:

1. In a blender or food processor, pulse to combine the watermelon, onion, cilantro, jalapeño, and lime juice only long enough to break down the Ingredients, leaving them very finely diced and taking care to not over process.

2. Pour into 1 large or 2 small bowls and enjoy.

Nutrition:

Calories: 35

Carbohydrates: 12

Fat: .4 g

Roasted Carrot and Leek Soup

Preparation Time: 4 minutes

Cooking Time: 30 minutes

Servings: 3-4

The carrot, a root vegetable, is an excellent source of antioxidants (1 cup has 113 percent of your daily value of vitamin A) and fibre (1 cup has 14 percent of your daily value). This bright and colourful soup freezes well to enjoy later when you're short on time.

Ingredients :

- 6 carrots
- 1 cup chopped onion
- 1 fennel bulb, cubed
- 2 garlic cloves, crushed
- 2 tablespoons avocado oil
- 1 teaspoon sea salt
- 1 teaspoon freshly ground black pepper
- 2 cups almond milk, plus more if desired

Directions:

1. Preheat the oven to 400°F. Line a baking sheet with parchment paper.

2. Cut the carrots into thirds, and then cut each third in half. Transfer to a medium bowl.

3. Add the onion, fennel, garlic, and avocado oil, and toss to coat. Season with the salt and pepper, and toss again.

4. Transfer the vegetables to the prepared baking sheet, and roast for 30 minutes.

5. Remove from the oven and allow the vegetables to cool.

6. In a high-speed blender, blend together the almond milk and roasted vegetables until creamy and smooth. Adjust the seasonings, if necessary, and add additional milk if you prefer a thinner consistency.

7. Pour into 2 large or 4 small bowls and enjoy.

Nutrition:

Calories: 55

Carbohydrates: 12g

Fat: 1.5 g

Protein: 1.8 g

Creamy Lentil And Potato Stew

Preparation Time: 10 minutes

Cooking Time: 30 minutes

Servings: 4

This is a hearty stew that is sure to be a favourite. It's a one-pot meal that is the perfect comfort food. With fresh vegetables and herbs along with protein-rich lentils, it's both healthy and filling. Any lentil variety would work, even a mixed, sprouted lentil blend. Another bonus of this recipe: It's freezer-friendly.

Ingredients :

- 2 tablespoons avocado oil
- ½ cup diced onion
- 2 garlic cloves, crushed
- 1 to 1½ teaspoons sea salt
- 1 teaspoon freshly ground black pepper
- 1 cup dry lentils
- 2 carrots, sliced
- 1 cup peeled and cubed potato
- 1 celery stalk, diced
- 2 fresh oregano sprigs, chopped
- 2 fresh tarragon sprigs, chopped
- 5 cups vegetable broth, divided
- 1 (13.5-ounce) can full-fat coconut milk

Directions:

1. In a great soup pot over average-high hotness, heat the avocado oil. Include the garlic, onion, salt, and pepper, and sauté for 3 to 5 minutes, or until the onion is soft.

2. Add the lentils, carrots, potato, celery, oregano, tarragon, and 2½ cups of vegetable broth, and stir.

3. Get to a boil, decrease the heat to medium-low, and cook, stirring frequently and adding additional vegetable broth a half cup at a time to make sure there is enough liquid for the lentils and potatoes to cook, for 20 to 25 minutes, or until the potatoes and lentils are soft.

4. Take away from the heat, and stirring in the coconut milk. Pour into 4 soup bowls and enjoy.

Nutrition:

Calories: 85

Carbohydrates: 20g

Fat: 3g

Protein: 3g

Roasted Garlic And Cauliflower Soup

Preparation Time: 10 minutes

Cooking Time: 35 minutes

Servings: 1-2

Roasted garlic is always a treat, and paired with cauliflower in this wonderful soup, what you get is a deeply satisfy soup with savoury, rustic flavors. Blended, the result is a smooth, thick, and creamy soup, but if you prefer a thinner consistency, just adds a little more vegetable broth to thin it out. Cauliflower is anti-inflammatory, high in antioxidants, and a good source of vitamin C (1 cup has 86 percent of your daily value).

Ingredients :

- 4 cups bite-size cauliflower florets
- 5 garlic cloves
- 1½ tablespoons avocado oil
- ¾ teaspoon sea salt
- ½ teaspoon freshly ground black pepper
- 1 cup almond milk
- 1 cup vegetable broth, plus more if desired

Directions:

1. Preheat the oven to 450°F. Line a baking sheet with parchment paper.

2. In a medium bowl, toss the cauliflower and garlic with the avocado oil to coat. Season with the salt and pepper, and toss again.

3. Transfer to the prepared baking sheet and roast for 30 minutes. Cool before adding to the blender.

4. In a high-speed blender, blend together the cooled vegetables, almond milk, and vegetable broth until creamy and smooth. Adjust the salt and pepper, if necessary, and add additional vegetable broth if you prefer a thinner consistency.

5. Transfer to a medium saucepan, and lightly warm on medium-low heat for 3 to 5 minutes.

6. Ladle into 1 large or 2 small bowls and enjoy.

Nutrition:

Calories: 48

Carbohydrates: 11g

Protein: 1.5g

Beefless "Beef" Stew

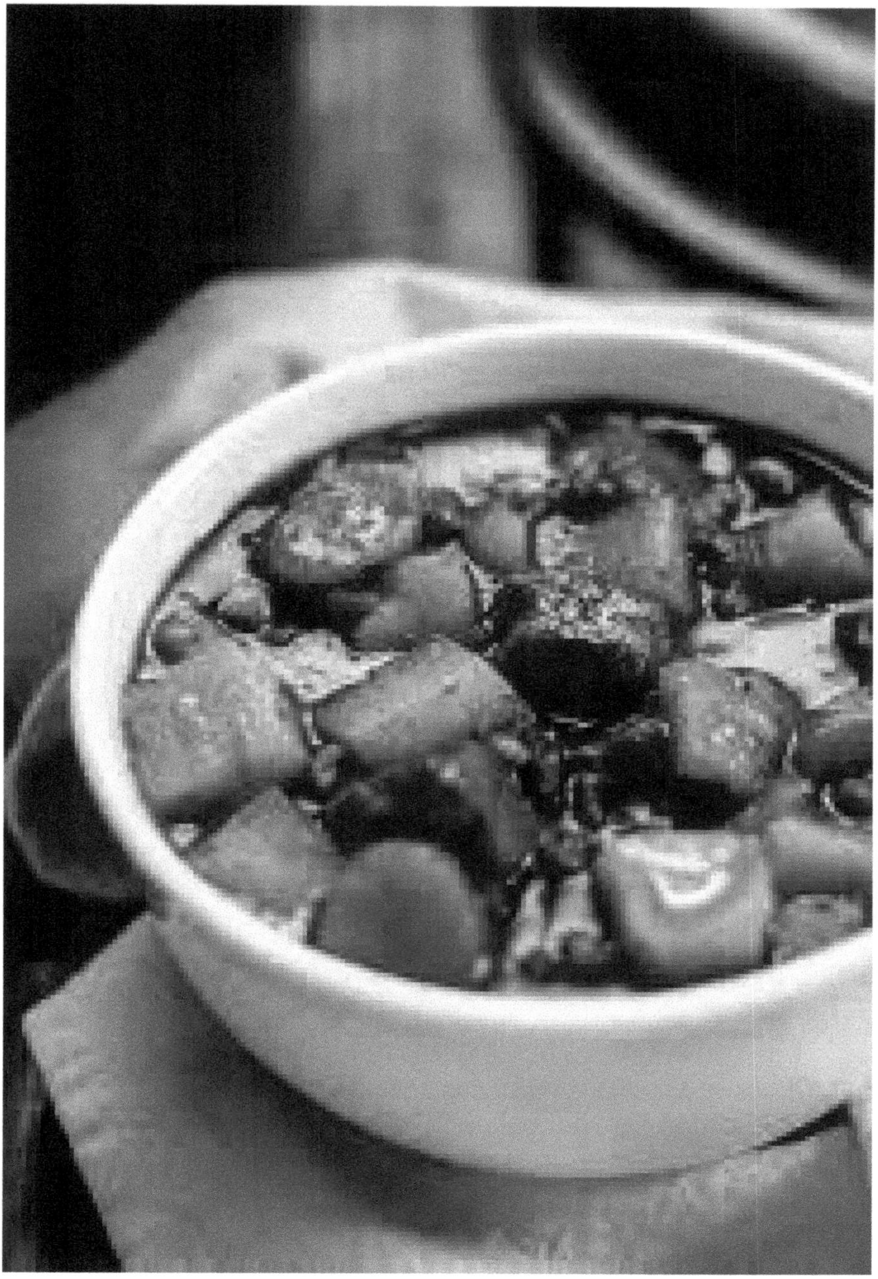

Preparation Time: 10 minutes

Cooking Time: 0 minutes

Servings: 4

The potatoes, carrots, aromatics, and herbs in this soup meld so well together, you'll forget there's typically beef in this stew. Hearty and flavourful, this one-pot comfort food is perfect for a fall or winter dinner.

Ingredients :

- 1 tablespoon avocado oil
- 1 cup onion, diced
- 2 garlic cloves, crushed
- 1 teaspoon sea salt
- 1 teaspoon freshly ground black pepper
- 3 cups vegetable broth, plus more if desired
- 2 cups water, plus more if desired
- 3 cups sliced carrot
- 1 large potato, cubed
- 2 celery stalks, diced
- 1 teaspoon dried oregano
- 1 dried bay leaf

Directions:

1. In a medium soup pot over medium heat, heat the avocado oil. Include the onion, garlic, salt, and pepper, and sauté for 2 to 3 minutes, or until the onion is soft.

2. Add the vegetable broth, water, carrot, potato, celery, oregano, and bay leaf, and stir. Get to a boil, decrease the heat to medium-low, and cook for 30 minutes, or until the potatoes and carrots be soft.

3. Adjust the seasonings, if necessary, and add additional water or vegetable broth, if a soupier consistency is preferred, in half-cup increments.

4. Ladle into 4 soup bowls and enjoy.

Nutrition:

Calories: 59

Carbohydrates: 12g

Creamy Mushroom Soup

Preparation Time: 5 minutes

Cooking Time: 20 minutes

Servings: 4

This savoury, earthy soup is a must try if you love mushrooms. Shiitake and baby Portobello (cremini) mushrooms are used here, but you can substitute them with your favourite mushroom varieties. Full-fat coconut milk gives it that close-your-eyes-and-savor-it creaminess that pushes the soup into the comfort food realm—perfect for those cold evenings when you need a warm soup to heat up your insides.

Ingredients :

- 1 tablespoon avocado oil
- 1 cup sliced shiitake mushrooms
- 1 cup sliced cremini mushrooms
- 1 cup diced onion
- 1 garlic clove, crushed
- ¾ teaspoon sea salt
- ½ teaspoon freshly ground black pepper
- 1 cup vegetable broth
- 1 (13.5-ounce) can full-fat coconut milk
- ½ teaspoon dried thyme
- 1 tablespoon coconut aminos

Directions:

1. In a great soup pot over average-high hotness, heat the avocado oil. Add the mushrooms, onion, garlic, salt, and pepper, and sauté for 2 to 3 minutes, or until the onion is soft.

2. Add the vegetable broth, coconut milk, thyme, and coconut aminos. Reduce the heat to medium-low, and simmer for about 15 minutes, stirring occasionally.

3. Adjust seasonings, if necessary, ladle into 2 large or 4 small bowls, and enjoy.

Nutrition:

Calories: 65

Carbohydrates: 12g

Fat: 2g

Protein: 2g

Chilled Berry And Mint Soup

Preparation Time: 5 minutes

Cooking Time: 20 minutes

Servings: 1-2

There's no better way to cool down when it's hot outside than with this chilled, sweet mixed berry soup. It's light and showcases summer's berry bounty: raspberries, blackberries, and blueberries. The fresh mint brightens the soup and keeps the sweetness in check. This soup isn't just for lunch or dinner either—tries it for a quick breakfast, too! If you like a thinner consistency for this, just add a little extra water.

Ingredients :

FOR THE SWEETENER

- ¼ cup unrefined whole cane sugar, such as Sucanat
- ¼ cup water, plus more if desired
- FOR THE SOUP
- 1 cup mixed berries (raspberries, blackberries, blueberries)
- ½ cup water
- 1 teaspoon freshly squeezed lemon juice
- 8 fresh mint leaves

Directions:

1. To prepare the sweetener

2. In a small saucepan over medium-low, heat the sugar and water, stirring continuously for 1 to 2 minutes, until the sugar is dissolved. Cool.

3. To prepare the soup

4. In a blender, blend together the cooled sugar water with the berries, water, lemon juice, and mint leaves until well combined.

5. Transfer the mixture to the refrigerator and allow chilling completely, about 20 minutes.

6. Ladle into 1 large or 2 small bowls and enjoy.

Nutrition:

Calories: 89

Carbohydrates: 12g

Fat: 6g

Protein: 2.2 g

Dill Celery Soup

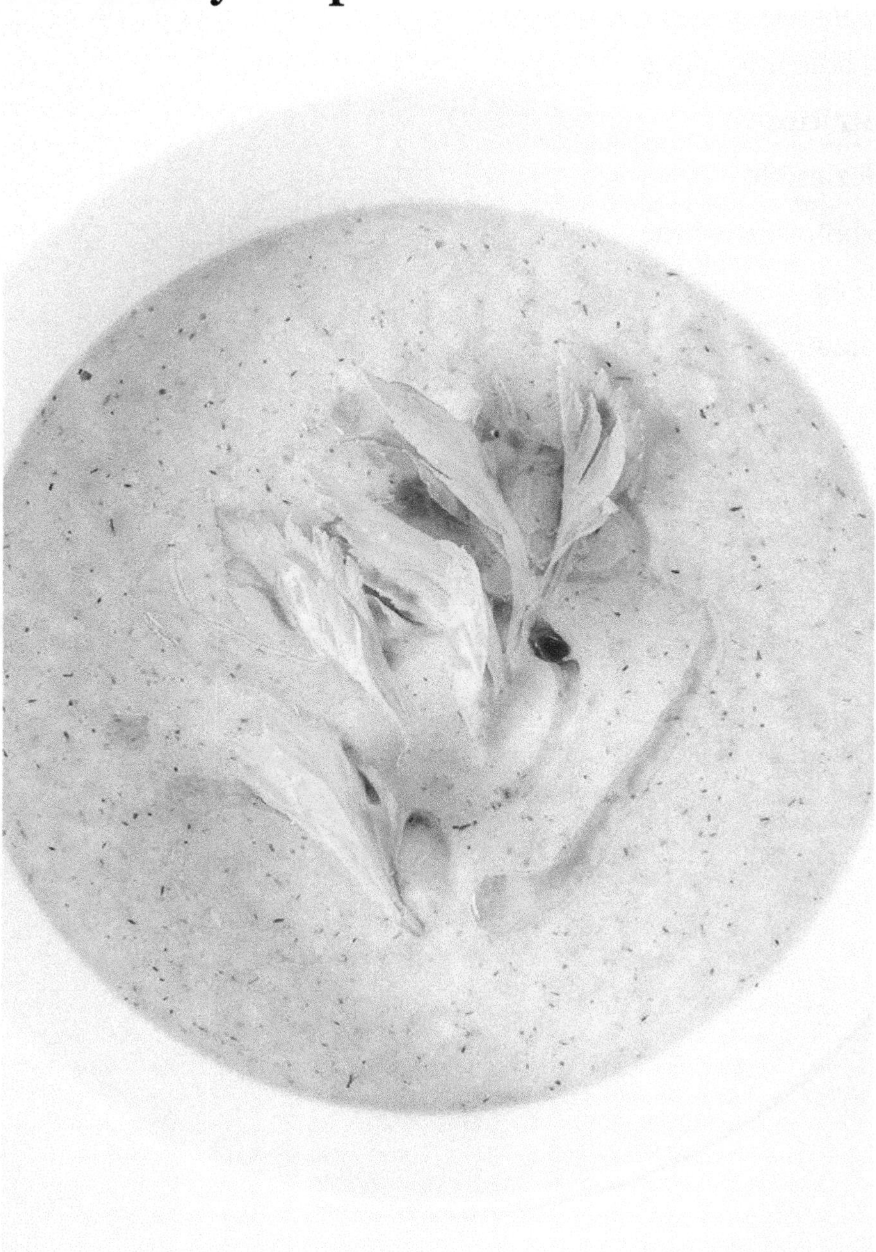

Preparation Time: 10 minutes

Cooking Time: 30 minutes

Servings: 4

Ingredients :

- 6 cups celery stalk, chopped
- 2 cups filtered alkaline water
- 1 medium onion, chopped
- 1/2 tsp. dill
- 1 cup of coconut milk
- 1/4 tsp. sea salt

Directions:

1. Combine all elements into the direct pot and mix fine.

2. Cover pot with lid and select soup mode it takes 30 minutes.

3. Release pressure using the quick release Directions: than open lid carefully.

4. Blend the soup utilizing a submersion blender until smooth.

5. Stir well and serve.

Nutrition:

Calories 193

Fat 15.3 g

Carbohydrates 10.9 g

Protein 5.2 g

Sugar 5.6 g

Cholesterol 0 mg

White Bean Soup

Preparation Time: 10 minutes

Cooking Time: 40 minutes

Servings: 6

Ingredients :

- 2 cups white beans, rinsed
- ¼ tsp. cayenne pepper
- 1 tsp. dried oregano
- ½ tsp. fresh rosemary, chopped
- 3 cups filtered alkaline water
- 3 cups unsweetened almond milk
- 3 garlic cloves, minced
- 2 celery stalks, diced
- 1 onion, chopped
- 1 tbsp. olive oil
- ½ tsp. sea salt

Directions:

1. Add oil into the instant pot and set the pot on sauté mode.

2. Add carrots, celery, and onion in oil and sauté until softened, about 5 minutes.

3. Add garlic and sauté for a minute.

4. Add beans, seasonings, water, and almond milk and stir to combine.

5. Cover pot with lid and cook on high pressure for 35 minutes.

6. When finished, allow to release pressure naturally then open the lid.

7. Stir well and serve.

Nutrition:

Calories 276

Fat 4.8 g

Carbohydrates 44.2 g

Sugar 2.3 g

Protein 16.6 g

Cholesterol 0 mg

Kale Cauliflower Soup

Preparation Time: 10 minutes

Cooking Time: 25 minutes

Servings: 4

Ingredients :

- 2 cups baby kale
- ½ cup unsweetened coconut milk
- 4 cups of water
- 1 large cauliflower head, chopped
- 3 garlic cloves, peeled
- 2 carrots, peeled and chopped
- 2 onion, chopped
- 3 tbsp. olive oil
- Pepper
- Salt

Directions:

1. Add oil into the instant pot and set the pot on sauté mode.

2. Add carrot, garlic, and onion to the pot and sauté for 5-7 minutes.

3. Add water and cauliflower and stir well.

4. Cover pot with lid and cook on high pressure for 20 minutes.

5. When finished, release pressure using the quick release Directions: than open the lid.

6. Add kale and coconut milk and stir well.

7. Blend the soup utilizing a submersion blender until smooth.

8. Season with pepper and salt.

Nutrition:

Calories 261

Fat 18.1 g

Carbohydrates 23.9 g

Sugar 9.9 g

Protein 6.6 g

Cholesterol 0 mg

Healthy Broccoli Asparagus Soup

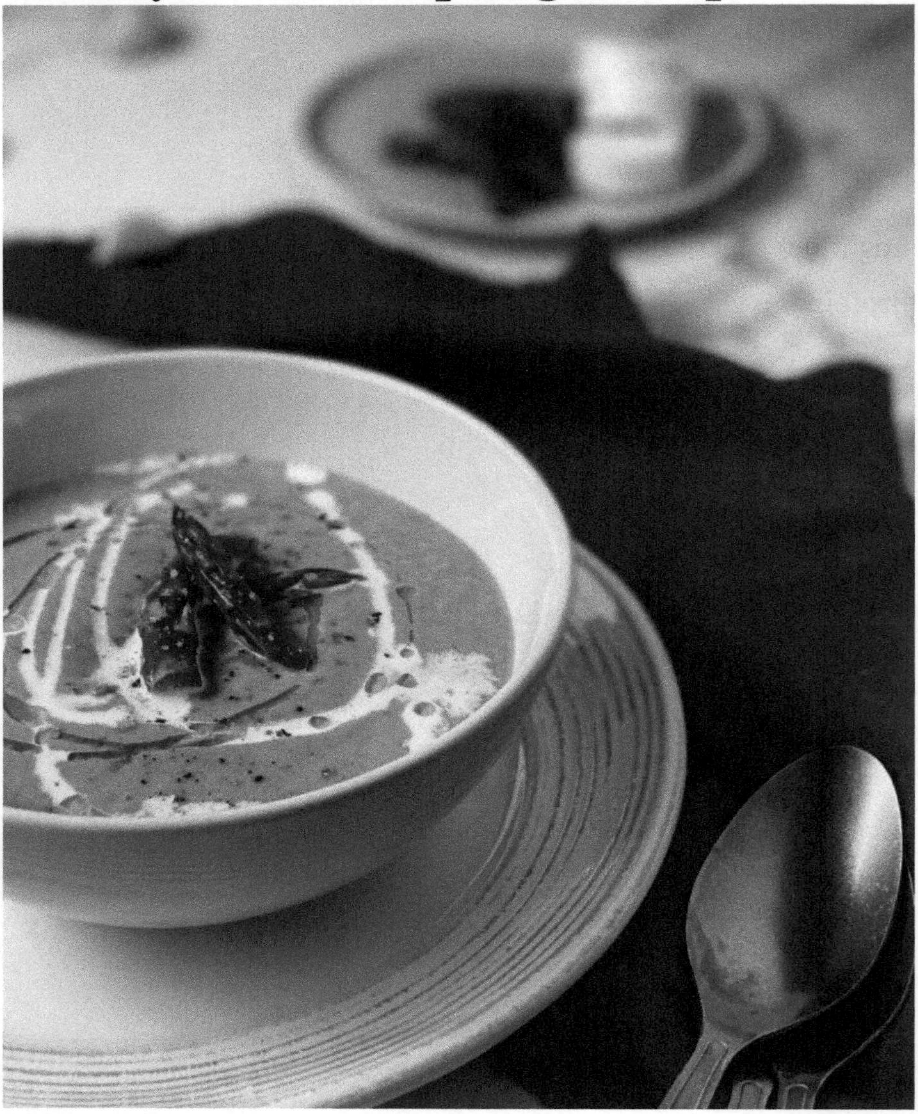

Preparation Time: 10 minutes

Cooking Time: 20 minutes

Servings: 6

Ingredients :

- 2 cups broccoli florets, chopped
- 15 asparagus spears, ends trimmed and chopped
- 1 tsp. dried oregano
- 1 tbsp. fresh thyme leaves
- ½ cup unsweetened almond milk
- 3 ½ cups filtered alkaline water
- 2 cups cauliflower florets, chopped
- 2 tsp. garlic, chopped
- 1 cup onion, chopped
- 2 tbsp. olive oil
- Pepper
- Salt

Directions:

1. Add oil in the instant pot and set the pot on sauté mode.
2. Add onion to the olive oil and sauté until onion is softened.
3. Add garlic and sauté for 30 seconds.
4. Add all vegetables and water and stir well.
5. Cover pot with lid and cook on manual mode for 3 minutes.
6. When finished, allow to release pressure naturally then open the lid.
7. Blend the soup utilizing a submersion blender until smooth.
8. Stir in almond milk, herbs, pepper, and salt.
9. Serve and enjoy.

Nutrition:

Calories 85

Fat 5.2 g

Carbohydrates 8.8 g

Sugar 3.3 g

Protein 3.3 g

Cholesterol 0 mg

Creamy Asparagus Soup

Preparation Time: 10 minutes

Cooking Time: 30 minutes

Servings: 6

Ingredients :

- 2 lbs. fresh asparagus cut off woody stems
- ¼ tsp. lime zest
- 2 tbsp. lime juice
- 14 oz. coconut milk
- 1 tsp. dried thyme
- ½ tsp. oregano
- ½ tsp. sage
- 1 ½ cups filtered alkaline water
- 1 cauliflower head, cut into florets
- 1 tbsp. garlic, minced
- 1 leek, sliced
- 3 tbsp. coconut oil
- Pinch of Himalayan salt

Directions:

1. Preheat the oven to 400 F/ 200 C.

2. Line baking tray with parchment paper and set aside.

3. Arrange asparagus spears on a baking tray. Drizzle with 2 tablespoons of coconut oil and sprinkle with salt, thyme, oregano, and sage.

4. Bake in preheated oven for 20-25 minutes.

5. Add remaining oil in the instant pot and set the pot on sauté mode.

6. Put some garlic and leek to the pot and sauté for 2-3 minutes.

7. Add cauliflower florets and water in the pot and stir well.

8. Cover pot with lid and select steam mode and set timer for 4 minutes.

9. When finished, release pressure using the quick release Directions.

10. Add roasted asparagus, lime zest, lime juice, and coconut milk and stir well.

11. Blend the soup utilizing a submersion blender until smooth.

12. Serve and enjoy.

Nutrition:

Calories 265

Fat 22.9 g

Carbohydrates 14.7 g

Sugar 6.7 g

Protein 6.1 g

Cholesterol 0 mg

Quick Broccoli Soup

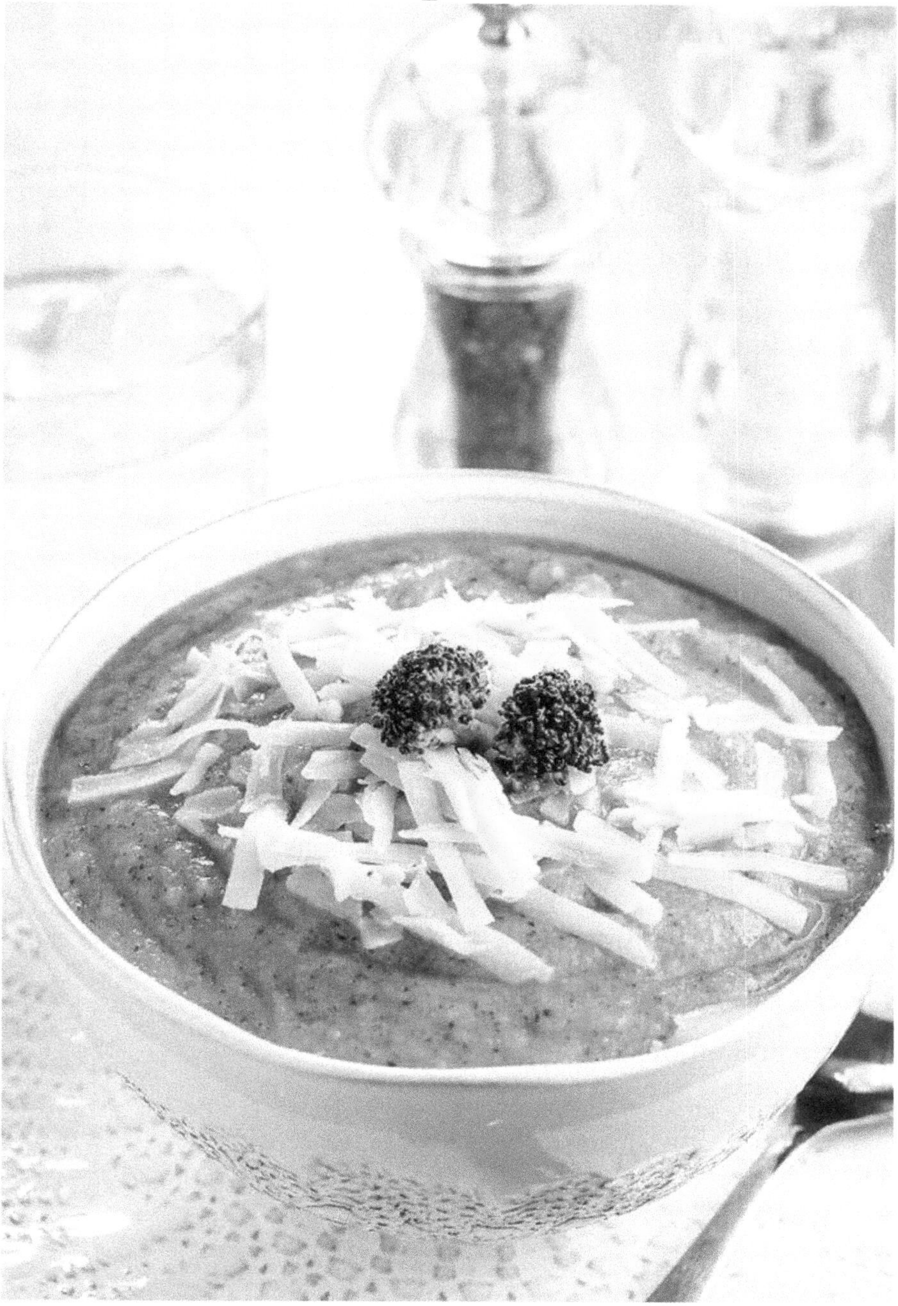

Preparation Time: 5 minutes

Cooking Time: 10 minutes

Servings: 6

Ingredients :

- 1 lb. broccoli, chopped
- 6 cups filtered alkaline water
- 1 onion, diced
- 2 tbsp. olive oil
- Pepper
- Salt

Directions:

1. Add oil into the instant pot and set the pot on sauté mode.

2. Add onion in olive oil and sauté until softened.

3. Add broccoli and water and stir well.

4. Cover pot with top and cook on manual high pressure for 3 minutes.

5. When finished, release pressure using the quick release Directions: than open the lid.

6. Blend the soup utilizing a submersion blender until smooth.

7. Season soup with pepper and salt.

8. Serve and enjoy.

Nutrition:

Calories 73

Fat 4.9 g

Carbohydrates 6.7 g

Protein 2.3 g

Sugar 2.1 g

Cholesterol 0 mg

Green Lentil Soup

Preparation Time: 10 minutes

Cooking Time: 30 minutes

Servings: 4

Ingredients :

- 1 ½ cups green lentils, rinsed
- 4 cups baby spinach
- 4 cups filtered alkaline water
- 1 tsp. Italian seasoning
- 2 tsp. fresh thyme
- 14 oz. tomatoes, diced
- 3 garlic cloves, minced
- 2 celery stalks, chopped
- 1 carrot, chopped
- 1 onion, chopped
- Pepper
- Sea salt

Directions:

1. Add all Ingredients except spinach into the direct pot and mix fine.

2. Cover pot with top and cook on manual high pressure for 18 minutes.

3. When finished, release pressure using the quick release Directions: than open the lid.

4. Add spinach and stir well.

5. Serve and enjoy.

Nutrition:

Calories 306

Fat 1.5 g

Carbohydrates 53.7 g

Sugar 6.4 g

Protein 21 g

Cholesterol 1 mg

Squash Soup

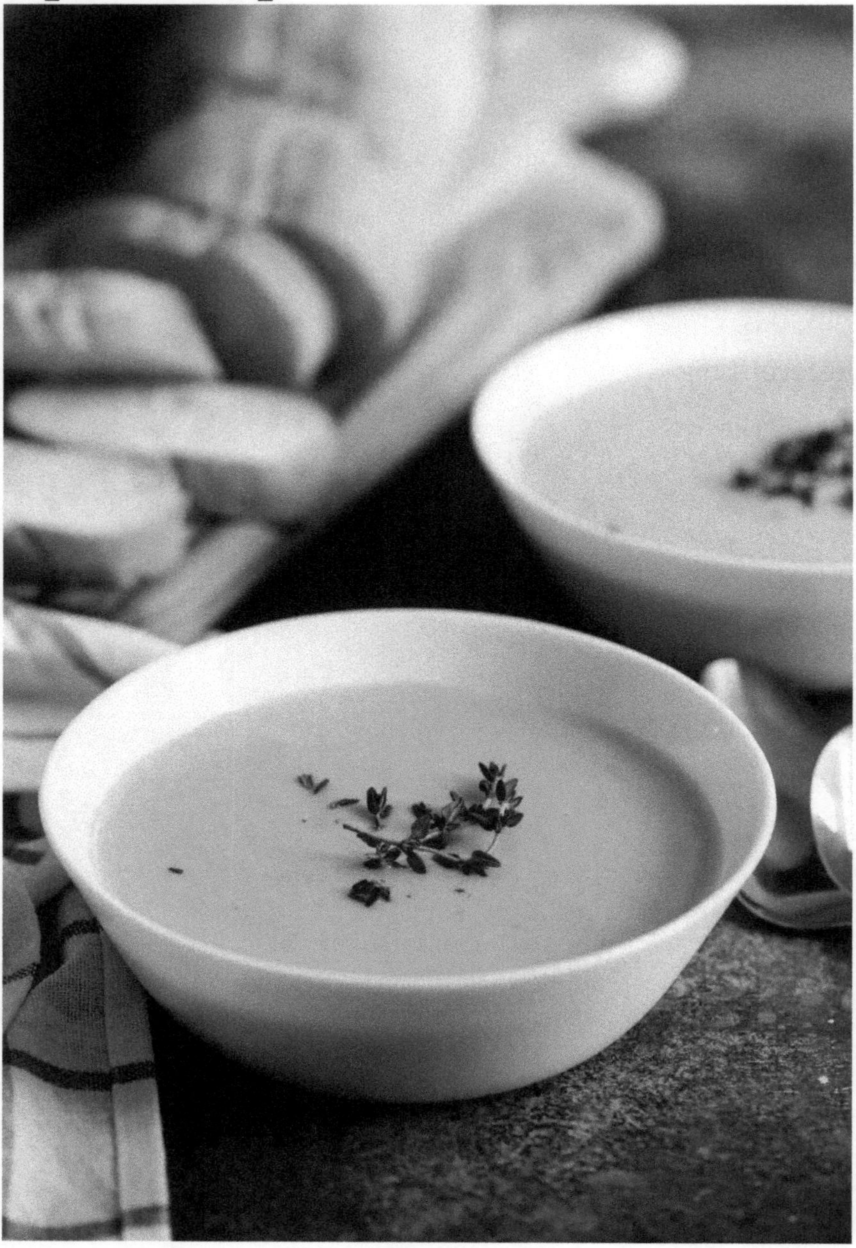

Preparation Time: 10 minutes

Cooking Time: 40 minutes

Servings: 4

Ingredients :

• 3 lbs. butternut squash, peeled and cubed

• 1 tbsp. curry powder

• 1/2 cup unsweetened coconut milk

• 3 cups filtered alkaline water

• 2 garlic cloves, minced

• 1 large onion, minced

• 1 tsp. olive oil

Directions:

1. Add olive oil in the instant pot and set the pot on sauté mode.

2. Add onion and cook until tender, about 8 minutes.

3. Add curry powder and garlic and sauté for a minute.

4. Add butternut squash, water, and salt and stir well.

5. Cover pot with lid and cook on soup mode for 30 minutes.

6. When finished, allow to release pressure naturally for 10 minutes then release using quick release Directions: than open the lid.

7. Blend the soup utilizing a submersion blender until smooth.

8. Add coconut milk and stir well.

9. Serve warm and enjoy.

Nutrition:

Calories 254

Fat 8.9 g

Carbohydrates 46.4 g

Sugar 10.1 g

Protein 4.8 g

Cholesterol 0 mg

Tomato Soup

Preparation Time: 5 minutes

Cooking Time: 20 minutes

Servings: 4

Ingredients :

- 6 tomatoes, chopped
- 1 onion, diced
- 14 oz. Coconut milk
- 1 tsp. turmeric
- 1 tsp. garlic, minced
- 1/4 cup cilantro, chopped
- 1/2 tsp. cayenne pepper
- 1 tsp. ginger, minced
- 1/2 tsp. sea salt

Directions:

1. Add all Ingredients to the direct pot and mix fine.

2. Cover instant pot with lid and cook on manual high pressure for 5 minutes.

3. When finished, allow to release pressure naturally for 10 minutes then release using the quick release Directions

4. Blend the soup utilizing a submersion blender until smooth.

5. Stir well and serve.

Nutrition:

Calories 81

Fat 3.5 g

Carbohydrates 11.6 g

Sugar 6.1 g

Protein 2.5 g

Cholesterol 0 mg

Summer Vegetable Soup

Preparation Time: 5 minutes

Cooking Time: 20 minutes

Servings: 10

Ingredients :

- 1/2 cup basil, chopped
- 2 bell peppers, seeded and sliced
- 1/ cup green beans, trimmed and cut into pieces
- 8 cups filtered alkaline water
- 1 medium summer squash, sliced
- 1 medium zucchini, sliced
- 2 large tomatoes, sliced
- 1 small eggplant, sliced
- 6 garlic cloves, smashed
- 1 medium onion, diced
- Pepper
- Salt

Directions:

1. Combine all elements into the direct pot and mix fine.

2. Cover pot with lid and cook on soup mode for 10 minutes.

3. Release pressure using quick release Directions than open the lid.

4. Blend the soup utilizing a submersion blender until smooth.

5. Serve and enjoy.

Nutrition:

Calories 84

Fat 1.6 g

Carbohydrates 12.8 g

Protein 6.1 g

Sugar 6.1 g

Cholesterol 0 mg

Almond-Red Bell Pepper Dip

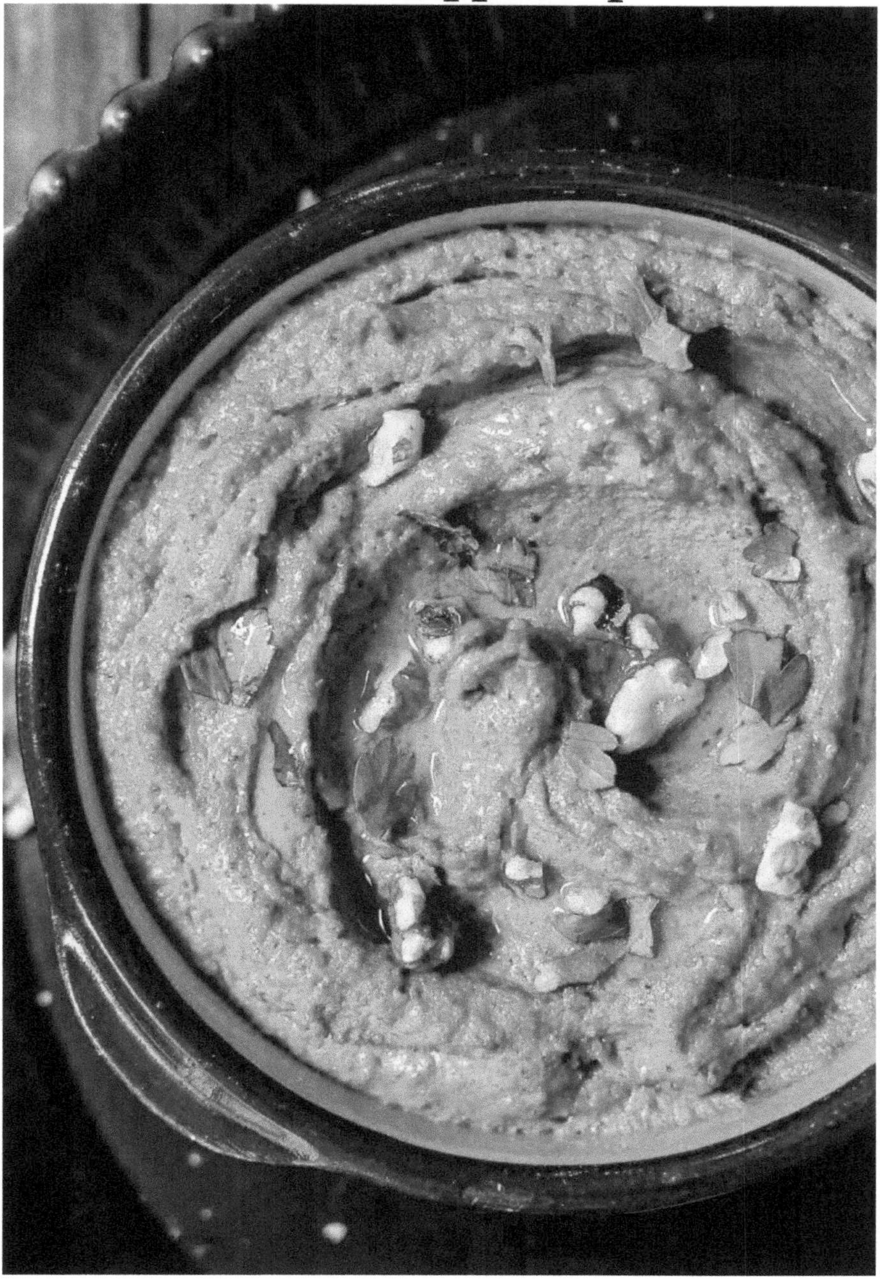

Preparation Time: 14 minutes

Cooking Time: 16 minutes

Servings: 3

Ingredients :

- Garlic, 2-3 cloves
- Sea salt, one (1) pinch
- Cayenne pepper, one (1) pinch
- Extra virgin olive oil (cold pressed), one (1) tablespoon
- Almonds, 60g
- Red bell pepper, 280g

Directions:

1. First of all, cook garlic and pepper until they are soft.

2. Add all Ingredients in a mixer and blend until the mix becomes smooth and creamy.

3. Finally, add pepper and salt to taste.

4. Serve.

Nutrition:

Calories: 51

Carbohydrates: 10g

Fat: 1g

Protein: 2g

Spicy Carrot Soup

Preparation Time: 10 minutes

Cooking Time: 20 minutes

Servings: 6

Ingredients :

- 8 large carrots, peeled and chopped
- 1 1/2 cups filtered alkaline water
- 14 oz. coconut milk
- 3 garlic cloves, peeled
- 1 tbsp. red curry paste
- 1/4 cup olive oil
- 1 onion, chopped
- Salt

Directions:

1. Combine all elements into the direct pot and mix fine.

2. Cover pot with lid and select manual and set timer for 15 minutes.

3. Allow to release pressure naturally then open the lid.

4. Blend the soup utilizing a submersion blender until smooth.

5. Serve and enjoy.

Nutrition:

Calories 267

Fat 22 g

Carbohydrates 13 g

Protein 4 g

Sugar 5 g

Cholesterol 20 mg

Raw Some Gazpacho Soup

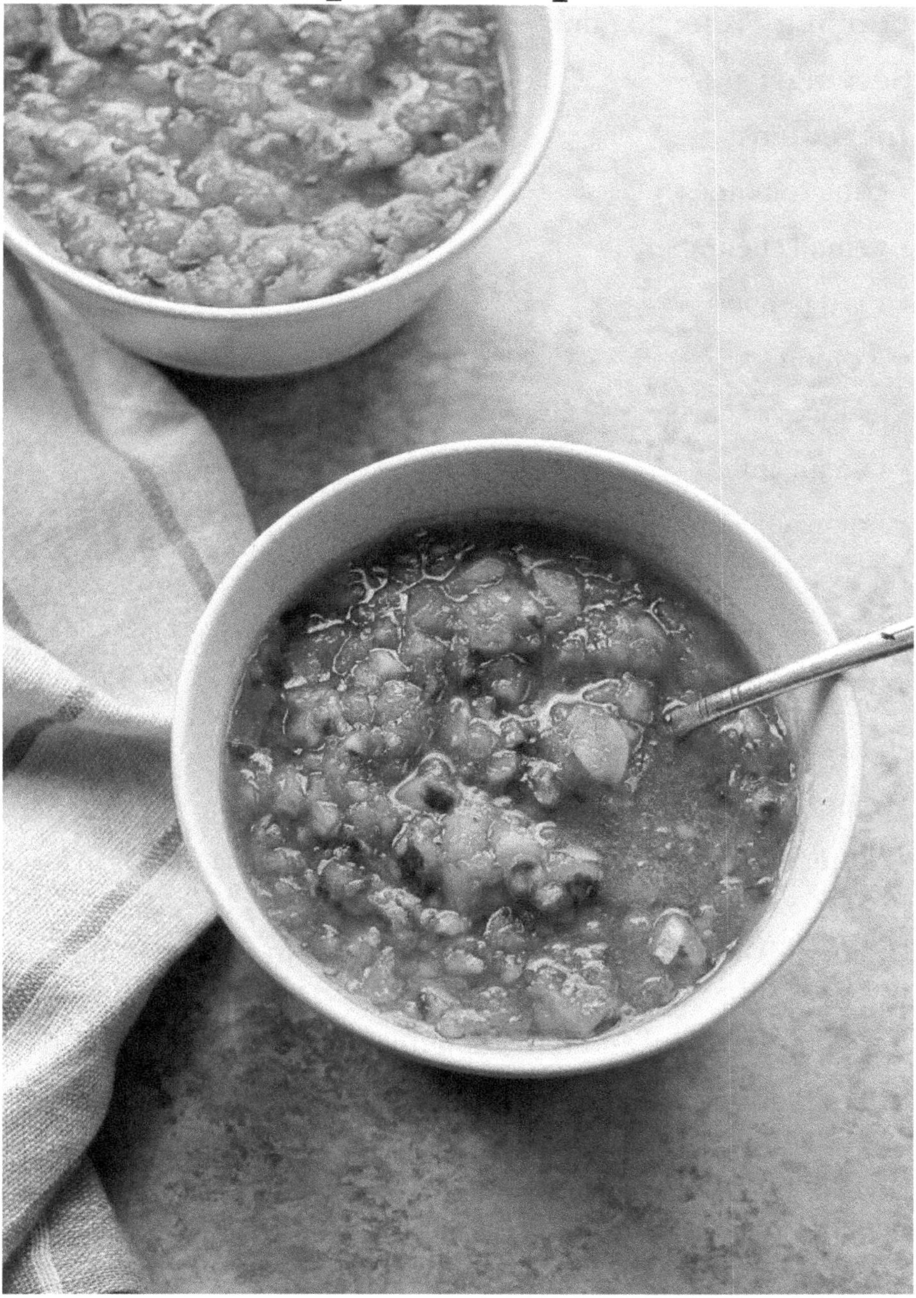

Preparation Time: 7 minutes

Cooking Time: 30 minutes

Servings: 3-4

Ingredients :

- 500g tomatoes
- 1 small cucumber
- 1 red pepper
- 1 onion
- 2 cloves of garlic
- 1 small chili
- 1 quart of water (preferably alkaline water)
- 4 tbsp. cold-pressed olive oil
- Juice of one fresh lemon
- 1 dash of cayenne pepper
- Sea salt to taste

Directions:

1. Remove the skin of the cucumber and cut all vegetables in large pieces.

2. Put all **Ingredients** except the olive oil in a blender and mix until smooth.

3. Add the olive oil and mix again until oil is emulsified.

4. Put the soup in the fridge and chill for at least 20 minutes.

5. Add some salt and pepper to taste, mix, place the soup in bowls, garnish with chopped scallions, cucumbers, tomatoes and peppers and enjoy!

Nutrition:

Calories: 39

Carbohydrates: 8g

Fat: 0.5 g

Protein: 0.2g

Alkaline Carrot Soup with Fresh Mushrooms

Preparation Time: 10 minutes

Cooking Time: 20 minutes

Servings: 1-2

Ingredients :

• 4 mid-sized carrots

• 4 mid-sized potatoes

• 10 enormous new mushrooms (champignons or chanterelles)

• 1/2 white onion

• 2 tbsp. olive oil (cold squeezed, additional virgin)

• 3 cups vegetable stock

• 2 tbsp. parsley, new and cleaved

• Salt and new white pepper

Directions:

1. Wash and strip carrots and potatoes and dice them.

2. Warm up vegetable stock in a pot on medium heat. Cook carrots and potatoes for around 15 minutes. Meanwhile finely shape onion and braise them in a container with olive oil for around 3 minutes.

3. Wash mushrooms, slice them to wanted size and add to the container, cooking approx. an additional 5 minutes, blending at times. Blend carrots, vegetable stock and potatoes, and put substance of the skillet into pot.

4. When nearly done, season with parsley, salt and pepper and serve hot. Appreciate this alkalizing soup!

Nutrition:

Calories: 75

Carbohydrates: 13g

Fat: 1.8g

Protein: 1 g

Swiss Cauliflower-Omental-Soup

Preparation Time: 10 minutes

Cooking Time: 15 minutes

Servings: 3-4

Ingredients :

- 2 cups cauliflower pieces
- 1 cup potatoes, cubed
- 2 cups vegetables stock (without yeast)
- 3 tbsp. Swiss Omental cheddar, cubed
- 2 tbsp. new chives
- 1 tbsp. pumpkin seeds
- 1 touch of nutmeg and cayenne pepper

Directions:

4. Cook cauliflower and potato in vegetable stock until delicate and Blend with a blender.

5. Season the soup with nutmeg and cayenne, and possibly somewhat salt and pepper.

6. Include emmenthal cheddar and chives and mix a couple of moments until the soup is smooth and prepared to serve. Enhance it with pumpkin seeds.

Nutrition:

Calories: 65

Carbohydrates: 13g

Fat: 2g

Protein: 1g

Chilled Parsley-Gazpacho With Lime & Cucumber

Preparation Time: 10 minutes

Cooking Time: 20 minutes

Servings: 1

Ingredients :

- 4-5 middle sized tomatoes
- 2 tbsp. olive oil, extra virgin and cold pressed
- 2 large cups fresh parsley
- 2 ripe avocados
- 2 cloves garlic, diced
- 2 limes, juiced
- 4 cups vegetable broth
- 1 middle sized cucumber
- 2 small red onions, diced
- 1 tsp. dried oregano
- 1½ tsp. paprika powder
- ½ tsp. cayenne pepper
- Sea salt and freshly ground pepper to taste

Directions:

1. In a pan, heat up olive oil and sauté onions and garlic until translucent. Set aside to cool down.

2. Use a large blender and blend parsley, avocado, tomatoes, cucumber, vegetable broth, lime juice and onion-garlic mix until smooth. Add some water if desired, and season with cayenne pepper, paprika powder, oregano, salt and pepper. Blend again and put in the fridge for at least 20 minutes.

3. Tip: Add chives or dill to the gazpacho. Enjoy this great alkaline (cold) soup!

Nutrition:

Calories: 48

Carbohydrates: 12 g

Fat: 0.8g

Chilled Avocado Tomato Soup

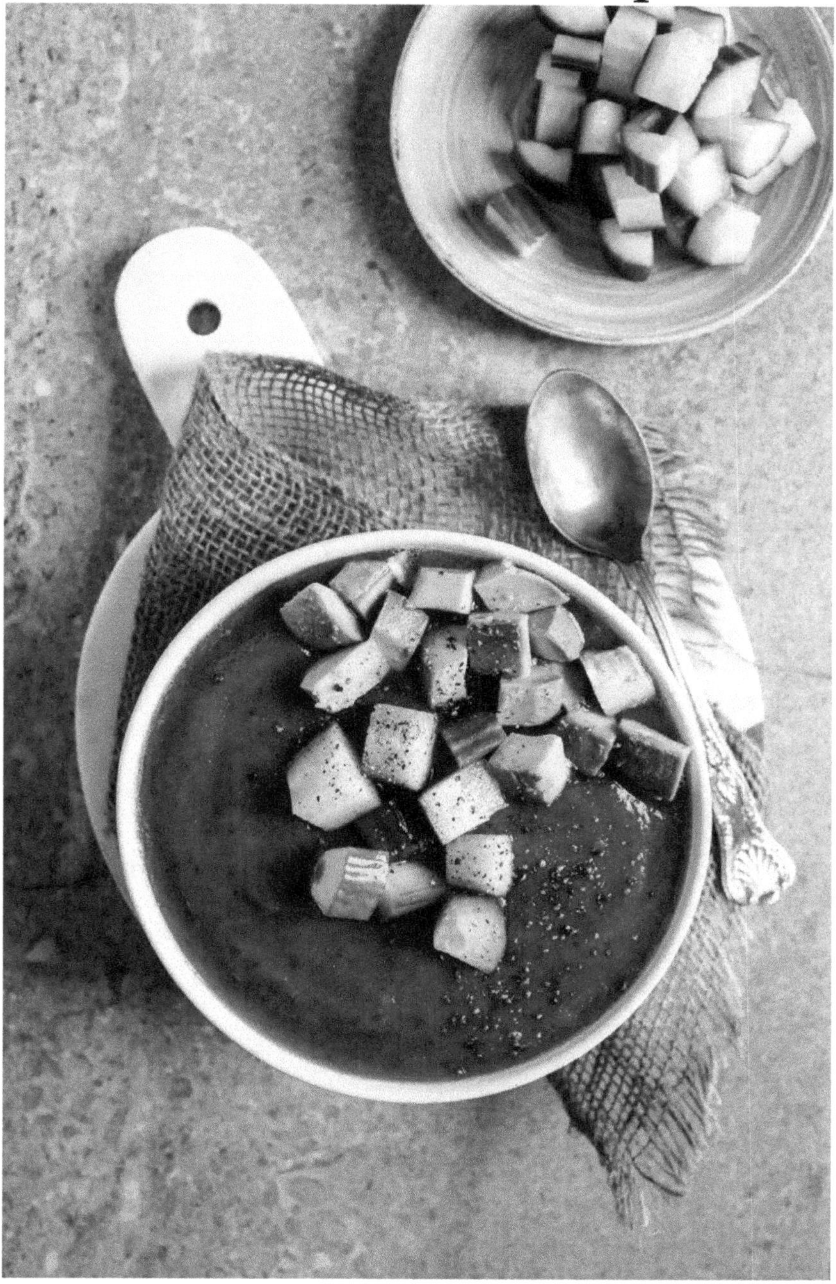

Preparation Time: 7 minutes

Cooking Time: 20 minutes

Servings: 1-2

Ingredients :

- 2 small avocados
- 2 large tomatoes
- 1 stalk of celery
- 1 small onion
- 1 clove of garlic
- Juice of 1 fresh lemon
- 1 cup of water (best: alkaline water)
- A handful of fresh lavage
- Parsley and sea salt to taste

Directions:

1. Scoop the avocados and cut all veggies in little pieces.

2. Spot all fixings in a blender and blend until smooth.

3. Serve chilled and appreciate this nutritious and sound soluble soup formula!

Nutrition:

Calories: 68

Carbohydrates: 15g

Fat: 2g

Protein: .8g

Pumpkin And White Bean Soup With Sage

Preparation Time: 10 minutes

Cooking Time: 40 minutes

Servings: 3-4

Ingredients :

- 1 ½ pound pumpkin
- ½ pound yams
- ½ pound white beans
- 1 onion
- 2 cloves of garlic
- 1 tbsp. of cold squeezed additional virgin olive oil
- 1 tbsp. of spices (your top picks)
- 1 tbsp. of sage
- 1 ½ quart water (best: antacid water)
- A spot of ocean salt and pepper

Directions:

1. Cut the pumpkin and potatoes in shapes, cut the onion and cut the garlic, the spices and the sage in fine pieces.

2. Sauté the onion and also the garlic in olive oil for around two or three minutes.

3. Include the potatoes, pumpkin, spices and sage and fry for an additional 5 minutes.

4. At that point include the water and cook for around 30 minutes (spread the pot with a top) until vegetables are delicate.

5. At long last include the beans and some salt and pepper. Cook for an additional 5 minutes and serve right away. Prepared!! Appreciate this antacid soup. Alkalizing tasty!

Nutrition:

Calories: 78

Carbohydrates: 12g

Alkaline Carrot Soup With Millet

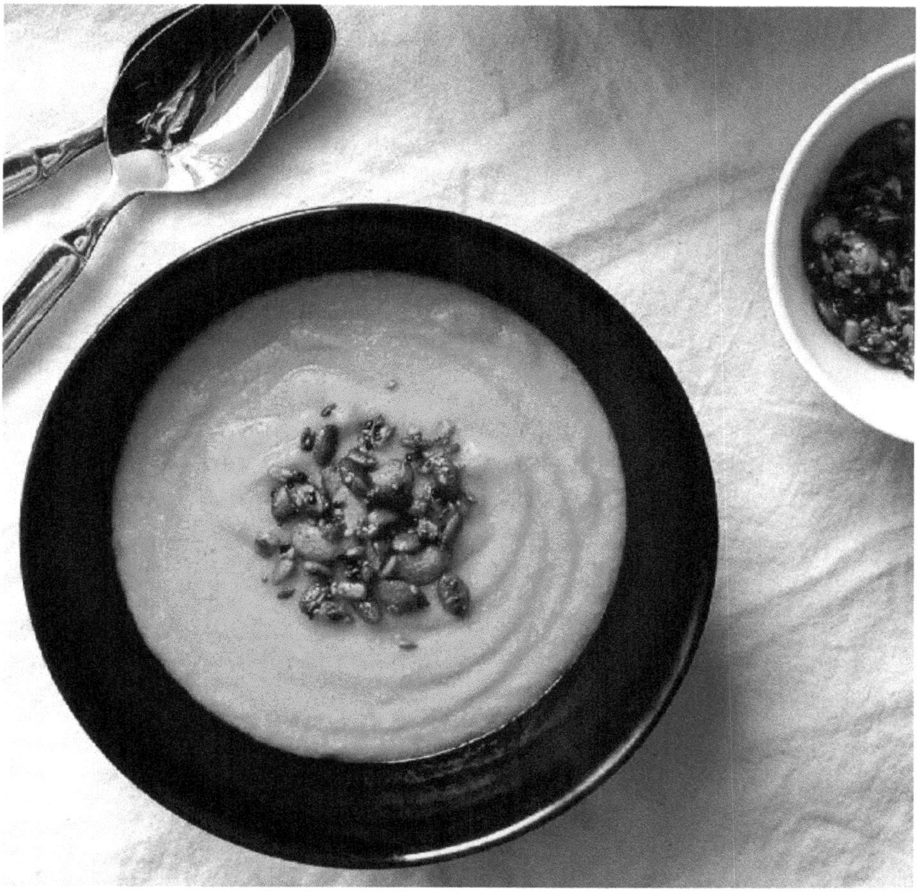

Preparation Time: 7 minutes

Cooking Time: 40 minutes

Servings: 3-4

Ingredients :

- 2 cups cauliflower pieces
- 1 cup potatoes, cubed

• 2 cups vegetables stock (without yeast)

• 3 tbsp. Swiss Emmenthal cheddar, cubed

• 2 tbsp. new chives

• 1 tbsp. pumpkin seeds

1 touch of nutmeg and cayenne pepper

Directions:

1. Cook cauliflower and potato in vegetable stock until delicate and Blend with a blender.

2. Season the soup with nutmeg and cayenne, and possibly somewhat salt and pepper.

3. Include emmenthal cheddar and chives and mix a couple of moments until the soup is smooth and prepared to serve. Can enhance with pumpkin seeds.

Nutrition:

Calories: 65

Carbohydrates: 15g

Fat: 1g

Protein: 2g

Alkaline Pumpkin Tomato Soup

Preparation Time: 15 minutes

Cooking Time: 30 minutes

Servings: 3-4

Ingredients :

- 1 quart of water (if accessible: soluble water)
- 400g new tomatoes, stripped and diced
- 1 medium-sized sweet pumpkin
- 5 yellow onions
- 1 tbsp. Cold squeezed additional virgin olive oil
- 2 tsp. ocean salt or natural salt
- Touch of Cayenne pepper
- Your preferred spices (discretionary)
- Bunch of new parsley

Directions:

1. Cut onions in little pieces and sauté with some oil in a significant pot.

2. Cut the pumpkin down the middle, at that point remove the stem and scoop out the seeds.

3. At long last scoop out the fragile living creature and put it in the pot.

4. Include likewise the tomatoes and the water and cook for around 20 minutes.

5. At that point empty the soup into a food processor and blend well for a couple of moments. Sprinkle with salt pepper and other spices.

6. Fill bowls and trimming with new parsley. Make the most of your alkalizing soup!

Nutrition:

Calories: 78

Carbohydrates: 20

Fat: 0.5g

Protein: 1.5g

Alkaline Pumpkin Coconut Soup

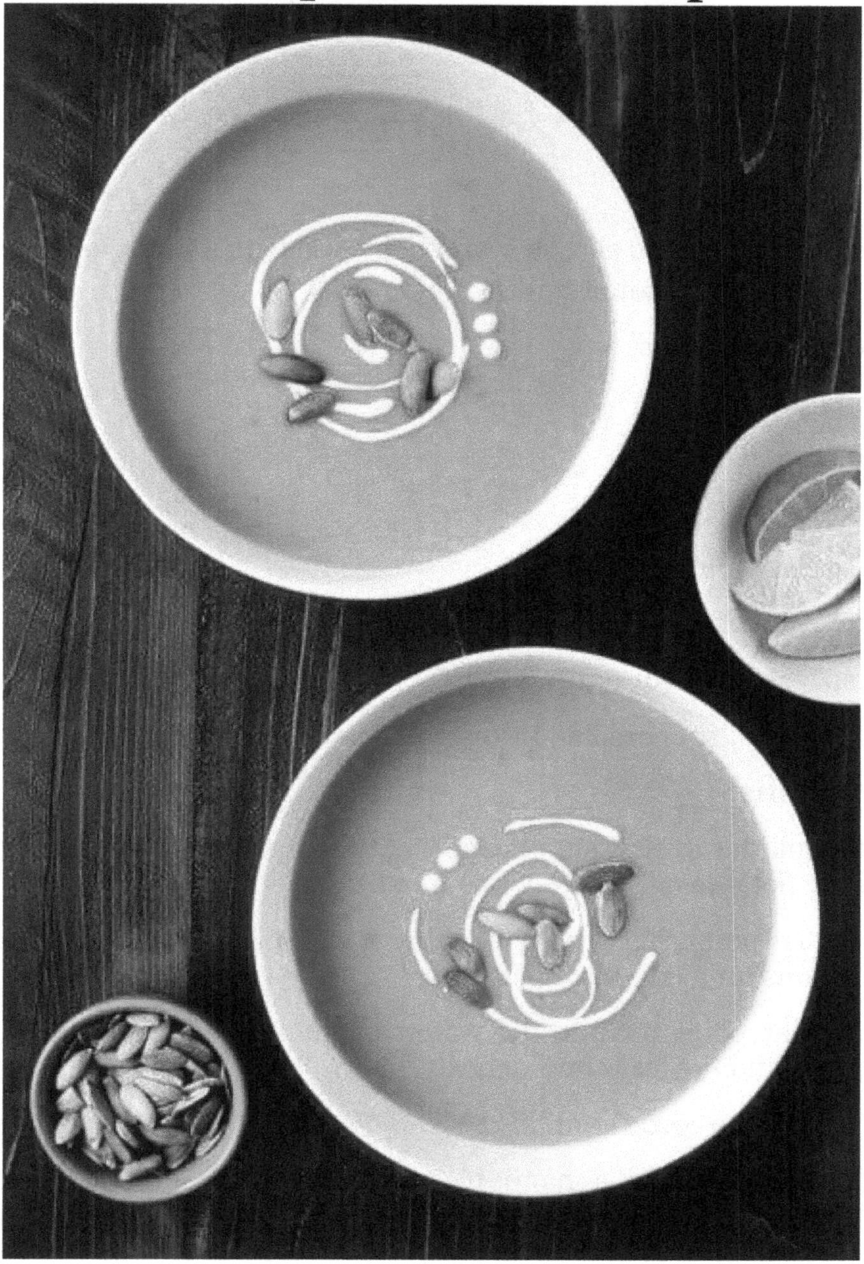

Preparation Time: 10 minutes

Cooking Time: 15 minutes

Servings: 3-4

Ingredients :

- 2lb pumpkin
- 6 cups water (best: soluble water delivered with a water ionizer) □ 1 cup low fat coconut milk
- 5 ounces potatoes
- 2 major onions
- 3 ounces leek
- 1 bunch of new parsley
- 1 touch of nutmeg
- 1 touch of cayenne pepper
- 1 tsp. ocean salt or natural salt
- 4 tbsp. cold squeezed additional virgin olive oil

Directions:

1. As a matter of first significance: cut the onions, the pumpkin, and the potatoes just as the hole into little pieces.

2. At that point, heat the olive oil in a significant pot and sauté the onions for a couple of moments.

3. At that point include the water and heat up the pumpkin, potatoes and the leek until delicate.

4. Include the coconut milk.

5. Presently utilize a hand blender and puree for around 1 moment. The soup should turn out to be extremely velvety.

6. Season with salt, pepper and nutmeg lastly include the parsley.

7. Appreciate this alkalizing pumpkin soup hot or cold!

Nutrition:

Calories: 88

Carbohydrates: 23g

Fat: 2.5 g

Protein: 1.8g

Cold Cauliflower-Coconut Soup

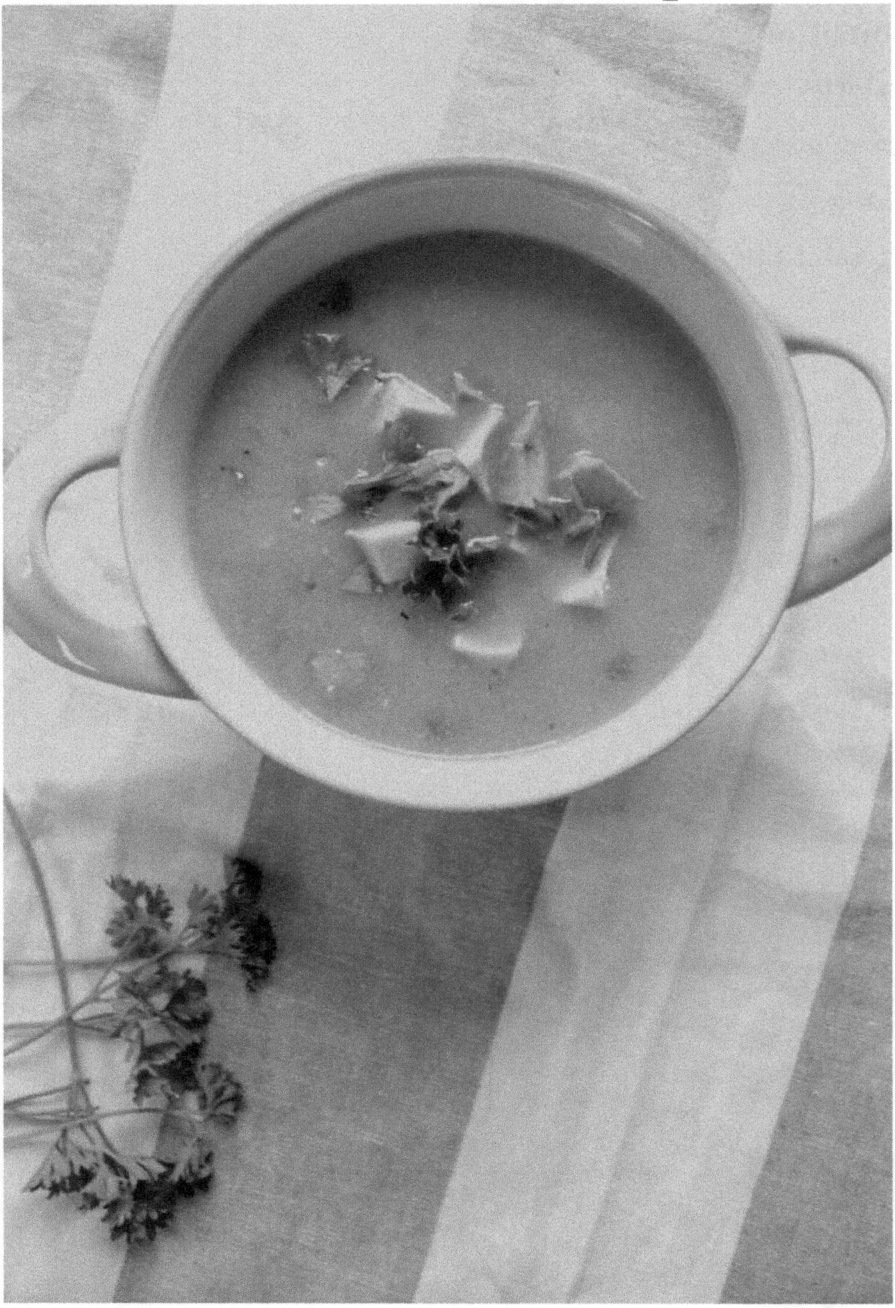

Preparation Time: 7 minutes

Cooking Time: 20 minutes

Servings: 3-4

Ingredients :

- 1 pound (450g) new cauliflower
- 1 ¼ cup (300ml) unsweetened coconut milk
- 1 cup water (best: antacid water)
- 2 tbsp. new lime juice
- 1/3 cup cold squeezed additional virgin olive oil
- 1 cup new coriander leaves, slashed
- Spot of salt and cayenne pepper
- 1 bunch of unsweetened coconut chips

Directions:

1. Steam cauliflower for around 10 minutes.

2. At that point, set up the cauliflower with coconut milk and water in a food processor and procedure until extremely smooth.

3. Include new lime squeeze, salt and pepper, a large portion of the cleaved coriander and the oil and blend for an additional couple of moments.

4. Pour in soup bowls and embellishment with coriander and coconut chips. Appreciate!

Nutrition:

Calories: 65

Carbohydrates: 11g

Fat: 0.3g

Protein: 1.5g

Raw Avocado-Broccoli Soup With Cashew Nuts

Preparation Time: 10 minutes

Cooking Time: 30 minutes

Servings: 1-2

Ingredients :

- ½ cup water (if available: alkaline water)
- ½ avocado
- 1 cup chopped broccoli
- ½ cup cashew nuts
- ½ cup alfalfa sprouts
- 1 clove of garlic
- 1 tbsp. cold pressed extra virgin olive oil
- 1 pinch of sea salt and pepper
- Some parsley to garnish

Directions:

1. Put the cashew nuts in a blender or food processor, include some water and puree for a couple of moments.

2. Include the various fixings (with the exception of the avocado) individually and puree each an ideal opportunity for a couple of moments.

3. Dispense the soup in a container and warm it up to the normal room temperature. Enhance with salt and pepper. In the interim dice the avocado and slash the parsley.

4. Dispense the soup in a container or plate; include the avocado dices and embellishment with parsley.

5. That's it! Enjoy this excellent healthy soup!

Nutrition:

Calories: 48

Carbohydrates: 18g

Fat: 3g

Protein: 1.4g

Alkaline Salsa Mexicana

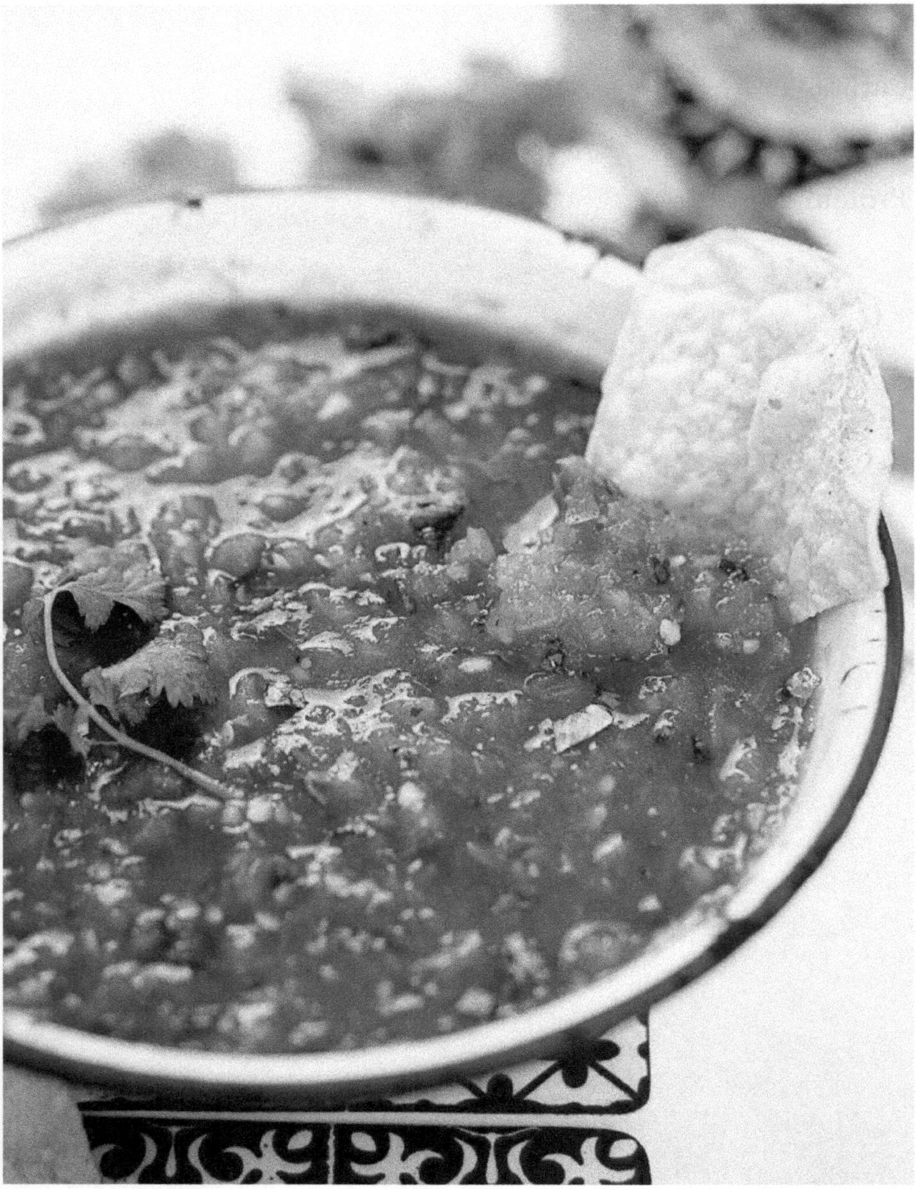

Preparation Time: 14 minutes

Cooking Time: 16 minutes

Servings: 3

Servings: one (1) bowl

Ingredients :

- Cayenne Pepper, one (1) pinch
- Spring onions, two (2)
- Tomatoes (big), three (3)
- Cilantro (a handful)
- Juice of lime, one (1)
- Organic or sea salt (one pinch)
- Chilies (green), two (2)
- Garlic, two (2) cloves

Directions:

1. Chop garlic cloves in tiny pieces, cut the chilies in small pieces, cut the onions in rings, and put the tomatoes in small cubes.

2. There are two ways you can about it, depend on how you prefer your salsa (either smooth or chunky).

3. For a smooth salsa; add all the Ingredients in a mixing pan and mix well.

4. Empty the mix in a food processor and blast for a few seconds.

5. Add salt and pepper to taste.

6. Serve.

7. However, for a chunky salsa; add all Ingredients together in a mixing bowl and mix properly.

8. Add salt and pepper to taste.

9. Serve.

Nutrition:

Calories: 5

Carbohydrates: 1g

Tofu Salad Dressing

Preparation Time: 14 minutes

Cooking Time: 16 minutes

Servings: 3

Ingredients :

- Stevia powder, One (1) teaspoon
- Tofu, 100g
- Alkaline water, Five (5) tablespoons
- Random spices and herbs of your choice
- Sea salt, ½ teaspoon

Directions:

1. Include all elements in a food processor and process until it is fine to consistency.

2. Enjoy it with salad.

Nutrition:

Calories: 80

Carbohydrates: 1g

Fat: 9g

Protein:1g

Millet Spread

Preparation Time: 14 minutes

Cooking Time: 16 minutes

Servings: 3

Ingredients :

- Pepper, one (1) pinch
- White onion (big), one (1)
- Millet, one (1) cup
- Any garden herb of your choice, one (1) teaspoon
- Virgin olive oil (cold pressed extra), one (1) tablespoon
- Alkaline water, two (2) cups
- Organic/sea salt, one (1) pinch
- Yeast free vegetable stock, one (1) teaspoon

Directions:

1. Get a small pot over medium heat, add water, the vegetable stock, and millet and boil for ten minutes, and put the pot aside for some minutes.

2. In a different pan, add oil and stir fry the roughly chopped onion.

3. Once that is done, add the stir-fried onion to the millet.

4. Mix properly, then add salt and pepper to taste.

5. Place it in a mixer and Blend for 40 seconds.

6. Serve.

Nutrition:

Calories: 25

Carbohydrates: 5 g

Alkaline Eggplant Dip

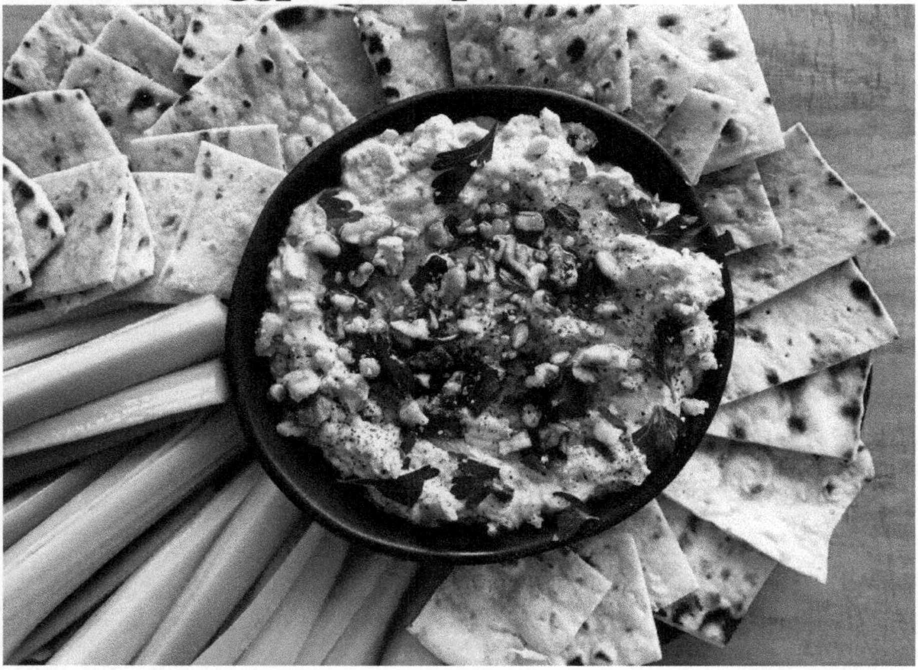

Preparation Time: 14 minutes

Cooking Time: 16 minutes

Servings: 3

Ingredients :

- Garlic, two (2) cloves
- Lemon juice (fresh), five (5) tablespoons
- Parsley (a handful)
- Cayenne pepper (a pinch)
- Organic salt or sea salt (a pinch)
- Eggplant (700g)
- Sesame paste, six (6) tablespoons

Directions:

1. Firstly, it is necessary to preheat the oven to around 400 degrees Fahrenheit.

2. Wash the eggplants and use a fork to prick several places.

3. Place in the oven on a grid and heat for between thirty to forty minutes.

4. While this is going one, chop the parsley and garlic and set aside.

5. Take off the eggplant from the oven after forty minutes and allow it to cool.

6. Once it's cooled, peel the eggplants and scoop out the pulp.

7. Chop the pulp finely on a chopping board and empty in a mixing bowl.

8. In the mixing bowl, sprinkle the lemon juice and mash with a spoon until it becomes smooth.

9. Finally, add garlic, the parsley, and the sesame paste.

10. Season with pepper and salt to taste.

11. Serve.

Nutrition:

Calories: 30

Carbohydrates: 2 g

Fat: 3 g

Protein: 1g

Coriander Spread

Preparation Time: 14 minutes

Cooking Time: 16 minutes

Servings: 3

Ingredients :

- Chili (green), 1-2
- Ginger (fresh), ½ inch
- Lime juice (fresh), two (2) tablespoons
- Coconut flakes (freshly grated), one (1) cup
- Coriander leaves (fresh), three (3) cups
- Alkaline water, four (4) tablespoons
- Organic or sea salt, one pinch

Directions:

1. Chop the ginger, chili and coriander leaves.

2. Include all elements in a blender machine and blend until the mix is smooth to consistency.

3. When that is done, you can add some organic or sea salt and season to taste.

4. Lastly, it is recommended that you put the mix in the fridge for about 35 minutes.

5. Serve.

Nutrition:

Calories: 22

Carbohydrates: 2 g

Fat: 43 g

Polo Salad Dressing

Preparation Time: 14 minutes

Cooking Time: 16 minutes

Servings: 3

Ingredients :

- Dates, two (2)
- Juice of lemon, (½ lemon)
- Alkaline water, ½ cup
- Cayenne pepper and sea salt, one (1) dash
- Extra virgin oil (cold pressed), 1/3 cup
- Miso, one (1) tablespoon

Directions:

1. Include all elements in a blender machine and blast until the mix is smooth to consistency.

2. You can add additional salt and pepper if desired.

3. Serve.

Nutrition:

Calories: 71

Carbohydrates: 8g

Fat: 3 g

Protein: 2g

Citrus Alkaline Salad Dressing

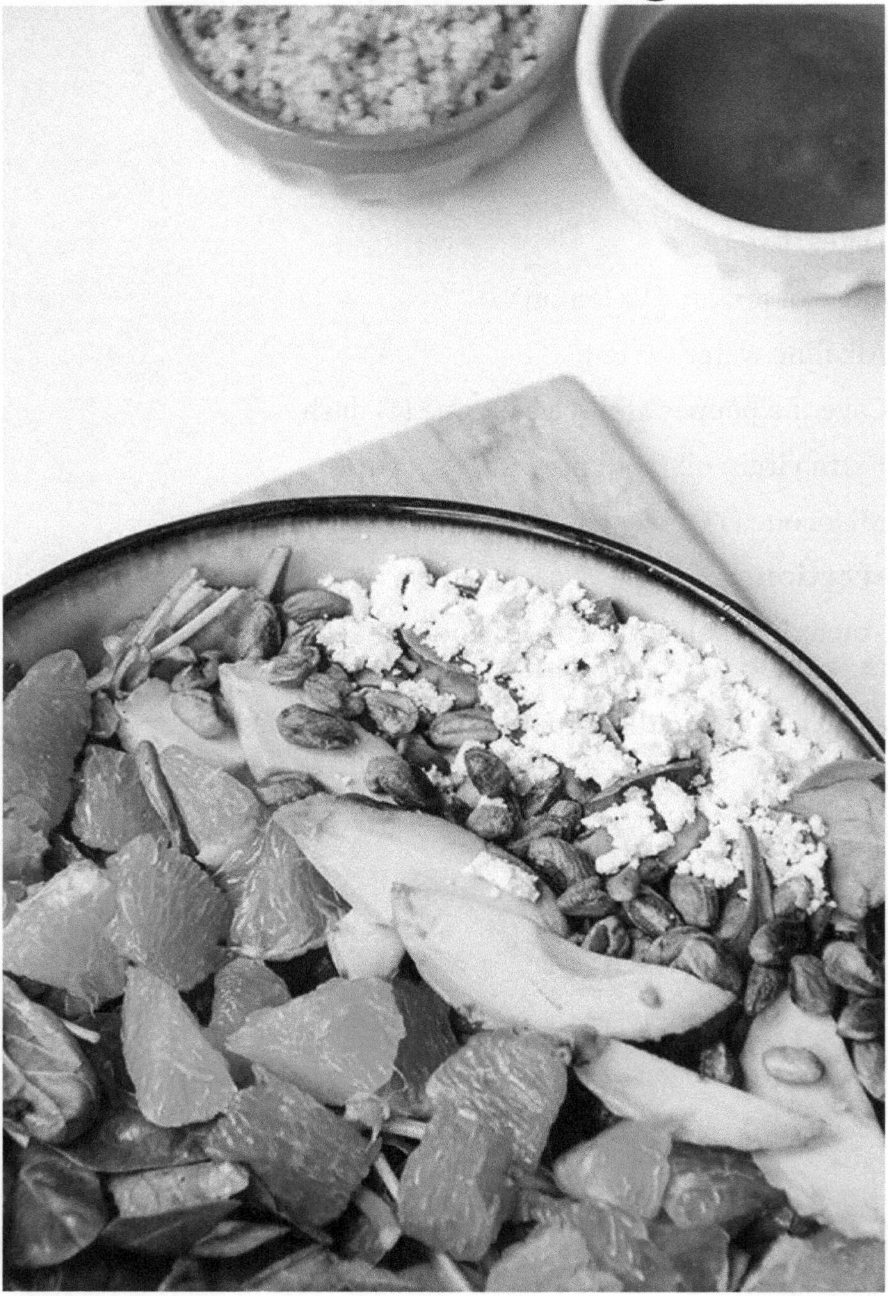

Preparation Time: 14 minutes

Cooking Time: 16 minutes

Servings: 3

Ingredients :

- Garlic powder, one (1) teaspoon
- Rosemary (dried), ¼ teaspoon
- Cumin (ground), ½ teaspoon
- Oregano (ground), ½ teaspoon
- Basil (dried), one (1) teaspoon
- Olive oil (cold pressed), ¾ cup
- Cayenne pepper and sea salt, one (1) dash
- Fresh lime or lemon juice, 1/3 cup

Directions:

1. Add all the Ingredients in a mixer and blast until the mix is smooth to consistency.

2. You can season with pepper and salt if desired.

3. Serve.

Nutrition:

Calories: 43

Carbohydrates: 3 g

Fat: 3 g

Avocado Spinach Dip

Preparation Time: 14 minutes

Cooking Time: 16 minutes

Servings: 3

Ingredients :

- Dill, one (1) cup
- Avocado, one (1)
- Garlic, one (1) clove
- Parsley, one (1) cup
- Spinach (fresh), 150g
- Tahini, one (1) tablespoon
- Chili, one (1)
- Pepper and sea salt to taste

Directions:

1. Include all elements in a blender machine

2. Blend until the mix turns creamy and smooth to consistency.

3. You can consist of pepper and salt to taste.

4. Serve.

Nutrition:

Calories: 46

Carbohydrates: 3g

Fat: 3g

Protein: 2g

Alkaline Vegetable Spread

Preparation Time: 14 minutes

Cooking Time: 16 minutes

Servings: 3

Ingredients :

- Pepper, one (1) pinch
- Tomato, one (1)
- Avocado, one (1)
- Yeast free vegetable stock, one (1) teaspoon
- Bean sprouts, ½ cup
- Celery stalk, one (1)
- Alfalfa sprouts, ½ cup
- Sunflower seeds, one (1) handful
- Organic salt or sea salt, one (1) pinch
- Any garden herb of your choice, one (1) teaspoon
- Extra virgin oil (cold pressed), one (1) tablespoon
- Cucumber ½

Directions:

1. Depending on how you like your spread, you can either Blend or not. Since we want this spread to be chunky, we won't Blend.

2. So, chop the alfalfa sprouts, cucumber, tomato, celery, and bean sprout into tiny pieces.

3. Get a mixing bowl and toss all the chopped Ingredients into it.

4. Add sunflower seeds and mix properly.

5. Mash the avocado and add in a separate bowl, along with the olive oil, vegetable stock, lemon juice, salt and pepper, and herbs.

6. Stir until it forms a creamy paste.

7. Finally, mix the mashed avocado cream with the vegetables.

8. Stir consistently until all Ingredients are mixed properly.

9. Refrigerate for about 35 minutes.

10. Serve.

Nutrition:

Calories: 12

Carbohydrates: 1 g

Fat: 7 g

Alkaline Sunflower Sauce

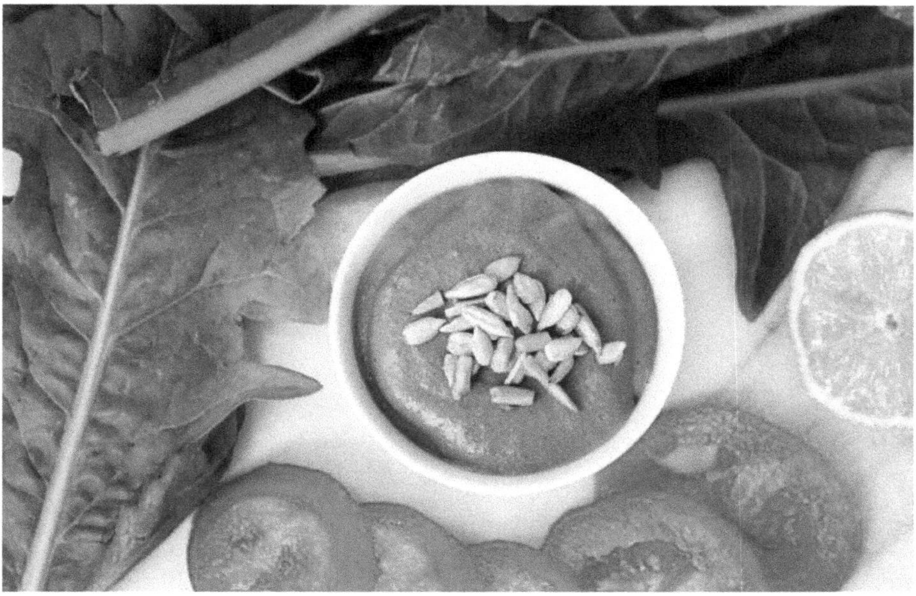

Preparation Time: 14 minutes

Cooking Time: 16 minutes

Servings: 3

Ingredients :

- Tomato, one (1)
- Sunflower seeds, 200g
- Red pepper, one (1)
- Garlic, one (1) clove
- Extra virgin olive oil (cold pressed), one (teaspoon)
- Pepper (a pinch)
- Organic salt or sea salt (a pinch)
- Any herb of your choice

Directions:

1. Note: Before you start this process, you should soak the sunflower seeds for about 40 minutes before commencement.

2. Add all Ingredients in a blender and blast till the mix turns into a smooth cream.

3. Add your favourite herbs, pepper and salt to taste.

4. Serve.

Nutrition:

Calories: 200

Protein: 7g

Hummus

Preparation Time: 14 minutes

Cooking Time: 16 minutes

Servings: 3

Servings: one (1)

Ingredients :

- Olive oil (cold pressed), one (1) tablespoon
- Fresh Lemon juice, two (2) tablespoons
- Chili, one (1)
- Pepper and sea salt to taste
- Tahini, one (1) tablespoon
- Garlic (finely chopped), two (2) cloves
- Chickpeas (home cooked), 300g-400g
- Vegetable broth (yeast-free), 50ml

Directions:

1. Blend all the Ingredients until it becomes creamy and smooth.

2. Add pepper and salt to taste.

3. Serve.

Nutrition:

Calories: 70

Carbohydrates: 4g

Fat: 5g

Protein: 2 g

Sweet Barbecue Sauce

Preparation Time: 14 minutes

Cooking Time: 16 minutes

Servings: 3

Ingredients :

- 6 quartered plum tomatoes
- 1/4 cup of chopped white onions
- 1/4 cup of date sugar
- 2 teaspoons of pure sea salt
- 2 teaspoons agave syrup
- 1/4 teaspoon cayenne
- 2 teaspoons of onion powder
- 1/2 teaspoon ground ginger
- 1/8 teaspoon cloves

Directions:

1. Add all ingredients, excluding date sugar, to a blender and blend them thoroughly. Pour mixture into saucepan and add a date sugar. Cook over average heat, stirring occasionally to prevent sticking until boiling. Reduce heat to a simmer. Cover the saucepan with lid and cook for 15 minutes, stirring from time to time.

2. Use an immersion blender to blend the sauce until it is smooth. Remain to cook at low heat until the sauce thickens for about 10 minutes. Allow mixture to cool before using. Serve and enjoy your Sweet Barbecue Sauce!

Nutrition:

Calories: 30

Carbohydrates: 4 g

Fat: 1 g

Avocado Sauce

Preparation Time: 14 minutes

Cooking Time: 16 minutes

Servings: 3

Ingredients :

- 1 ripe Avocado
- 1 pinch of Basil
- ½ teaspoon of Oregano
- 1/2 teaspoon of onion powder
- 2 teaspoons of minced onion
- 1/2 teaspoon of pure sea salt

Directions:

1. Cut the avocado in half, peel it and remove the seed. Slice it into small pieces and throw into a food processor.

2. Add all other Ingredients and blend for 2 to 3 minutes until smooth.

3. Serve and enjoy your avocado sauce!

Nutrition:

Calories: 14

Carbohydrates: 2 g

Protein: 1g

Fragrant Tomato Sauce

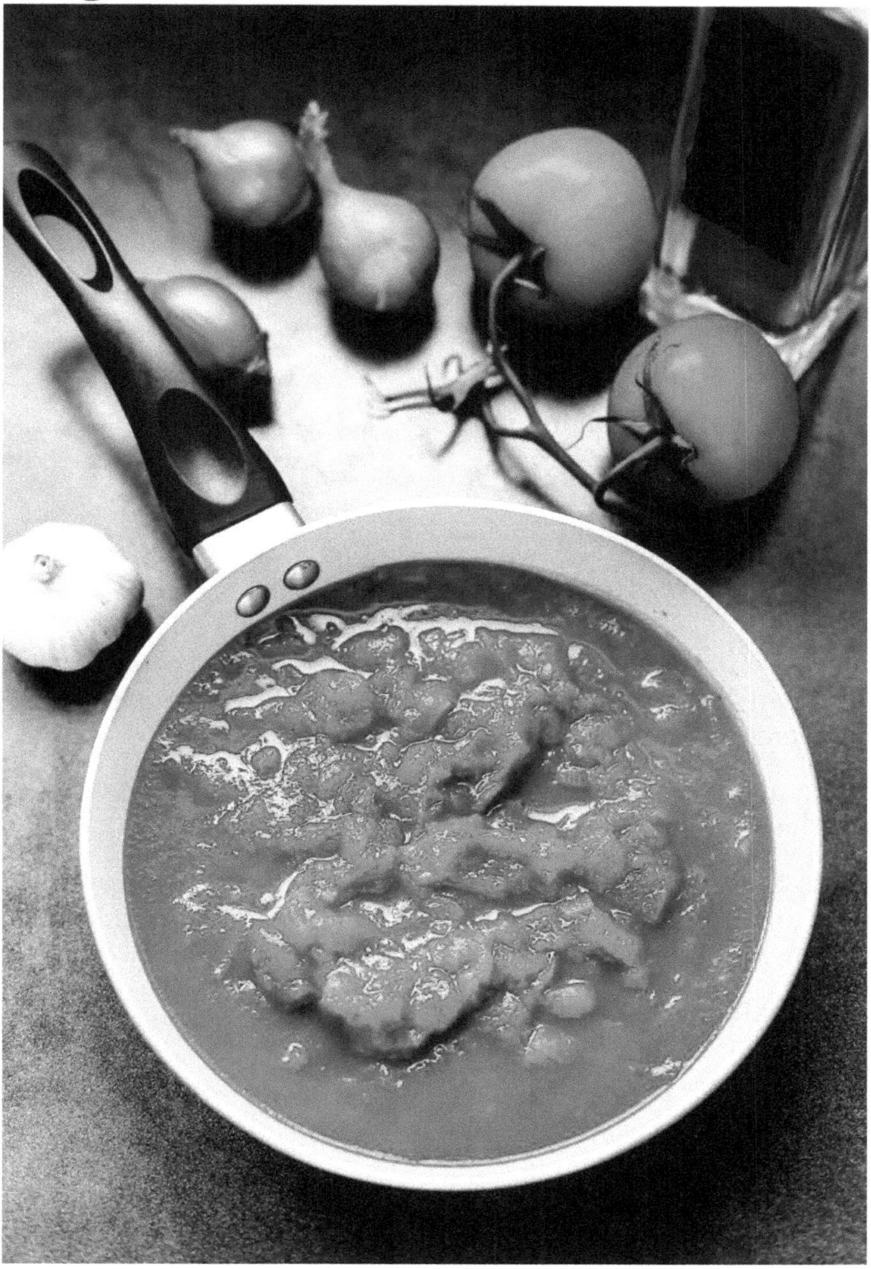

Preparation Time: 14 minutes

Cooking Time: 16 minutes

Servings: 3

Ingredients :

- 5 roma tomatoes
- 1 pinch of basil
- 1 teaspoon of oregano
- 1 teaspoon of onion powder
- 2 teaspoon of minced onion
- 2 teaspoon agave syrup
- 1 teaspoon of pure sea salt
- 2 tablespoons of grape seed oil

Directions:

1. Make an X cut on the lowermost of the Roma Tomatoes and place them into a pot of hot water for just 1 minute.

2. Take away the tomatoes from the water using a spoon and shock them, placing them in cold water for 30 seconds.

3. Take them out and immediately peel with your fingers or a knife. Put all the Ingredients into a mixer or a food processor and blend for 1 minute until smooth.

4. Serve and enjoy your fragrant tomato sauce.

Nutrition:

Calories: 20

Carbohydrates: 2 g

Protein: 1g

Guacamole

Preparation Time: 14 minutes

Cooking Time: 16 minutes

Servings: 3

Ingredients :

- 1 minced roma tomato
- 2 avocados
- 1/2 cup of chopped cilantro
- 1/2 cup of minced red onion
- 1/2 teaspoon of cayenne powder
- 1/2 teaspoon of onion powder
- 1/2 teaspoon of pure sea salt
- Juice from ½ lime

Directions:

1. Cut the avocados in half, peel and remove the seeds.

2. Slice into tiny pieces and put them in a medium bowl. Add all other Ingredients, excluding the roma tomato, to the bowl. Using a masher, mix together until becomes smooth.

3. Add the minced roma tomatoes to the mixture and mix well.

4. Serve and enjoy your delicious Guacamole!

Nutrition:

Calories: 12

Fat: 1 g

Garlic Sauce

Preparation Time: 14 minutes

Cooking Time: 16 minutes

Servings: 3

Ingredients :

- 1/4 cup of diced shallots
- 1 tablespoon of onion powder
- 1/4 teaspoon of dill
- 1/2 teaspoon of ginger
- 1/2 teaspoon of pure sea salt
- 1 cup of grape seed oil

Directions:

1. Find a glass jar with a lid. Put all Ingredients for the sauce in the jar and shake them well.

2. Place the sauce mixture in the refrigerator for at least 20 minutes.

3. Serve and enjoy your "Garlic" Sauce!

Nutrition:

Calories: 48

Carbohydrates: 2 g

Fat: 4 g

Pesto Saucy Cream Recipe

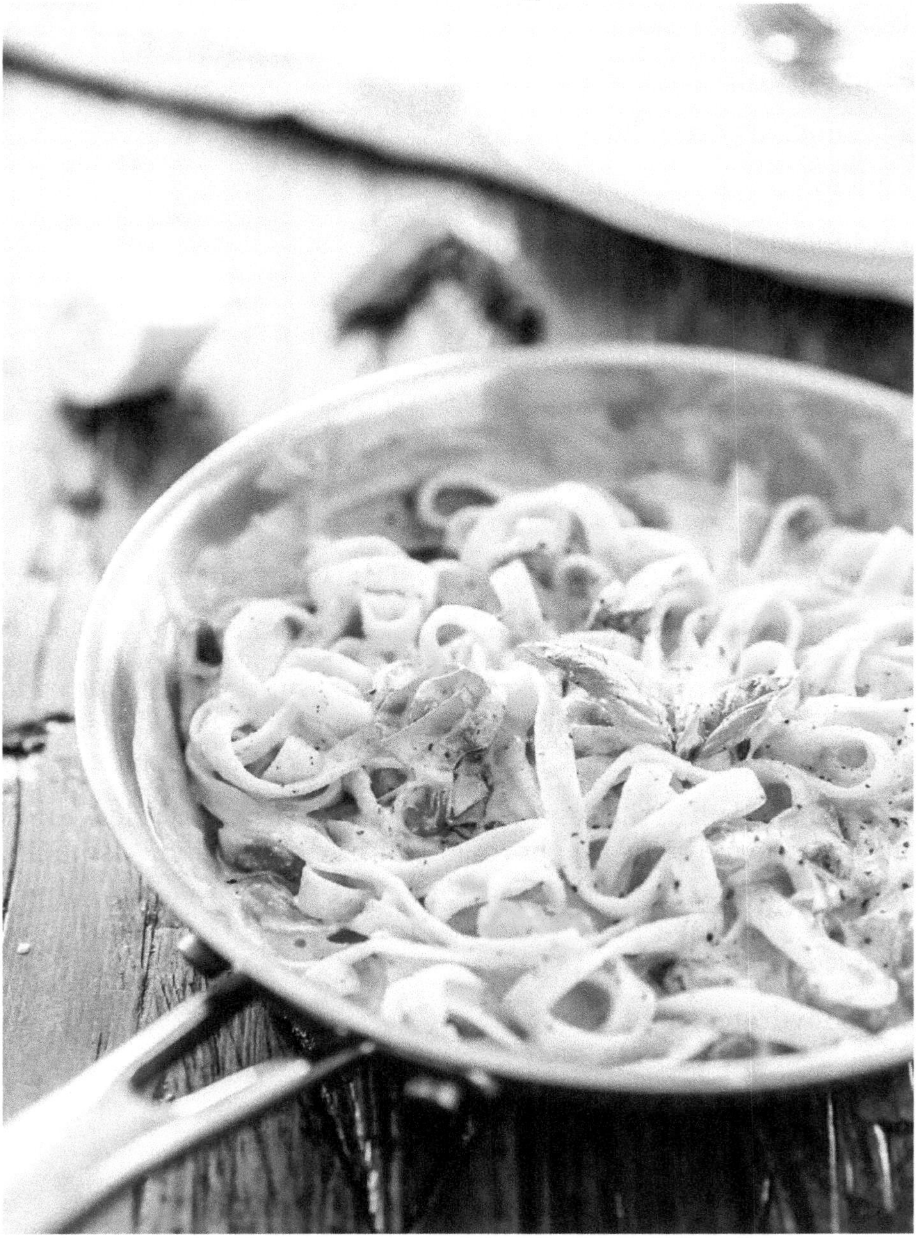

Preparation Time: 14 minutes

Cooking Time: 16 minutes

Servings: 3

Ingredients :

- 1 small avocado (hass)
- 1 cup walnuts
- 3 tablespoons sour orange or lime
- 1/8 teaspoon basil
- 1/4 teaspoon onion powder
- 1/4 teaspoon cayenne pepper
- 1 teaspoon spring water

Directions:

1. Make slit with knife length wise all the way round the avocado.

2. Split open the avocado into two.

3. Then using your heavy knife, carefully hit down the avocado seed, turn and pull out the seed. Scoop out the avocado meat and remove the skin.

4. Then, add all of the Ingredients to your blender and blend until all of the Ingredients are thoroughly mixed and becomes smooth.

Nutrition:

Calories: 65

Carbohydrates: 4 g

Fat: 5 g

Protein: 3 g

Lightning Source UK Ltd.
Milton Keynes UK
UKHW021227101022
410224UK00001B/17

9 781802 695120